ONE FOUR

BY JOY FORD

'One Million People Commit Suicide Every Year'
The World Health Organization

Published by:
Chipmunkapublishing
PO Box 6872
Brentwood
Essex
CM13 1ZT
United Kingdom

http://www.chipmunkapublishing.com

Acknowledgements
I wanted to write Edward's story for sometime, but it has taken a few years to collect my thoughts and wait for them to be rational, before I could begin. For a long time I wasn't sure how I could start, until a dear friend unknowingly gave me the beginning. All the events that take place in this book are true, but it is told only from my point of view, others who were there at the time may have a different prospective and can only remember things from their own point of view. I can not speak for them and have not tried to, we all have different realities and this is mine. Names have been changed apart from mine and my youngest child Edward.

This book has been possible, due to the support of many people, in many different ways. They have all helped me through my journey of Edward's illness and my grief at different times and enabled me to carry on with life.

Big thanks to Doctors Jill Kershaw, Sandra Wiltshire, and Harry Dickinson, for their support, empathy, and endless patience. You four showed me the way through the hell I felt I had fallen in when I was ready to give up.

Thanks to my brother Roy and Sandy his wife for always being there and keeping in touch especially in the beginning, you'll never know what those phone calls meant to me.

Big thanks to Jean Greco for always being at the

end of the phone, for your listening, understanding, and for giving up your time often at short notice, to be with me.

Thanks to Maureen and Ian George who had their own battle to fight, but took time to think of me and gave me the sanctuary of Corner Cottage, where I found peace in my heart again.

Thanks to Jan Kidd, Ginny Baker, Darrell Hebdon and Aide Fisher, four very special people, who put so much into helping others, for so little reward, you were all four brilliant. I felt it an honour to know you.

Thanks to James Sykes for all his help advice and support leading up to the inquest and after. You made a terrible ordeal bearable.

Thanks to all my family especially
Julia Best for her amazing support and love to us all one terrible Easter Monday.
Big thanks to Emma, for often putting her grief on hold to be there for me, I'm so lucky to have such a loving and generous daughter.
Biggest thanks to my husband who went through it all with me, for all his hugs, and his knowing when to say nothing, and when I needed him to talk to me. The past four years have been a roller coaster of emotions and you held me on that ride with love.

Thank to Marie Hughes for taking me to places and keeping me going, your laughter was infectious and I learnt to smile again.

Thanks to Spencer Baker who had the patience to listen to my demented phone calls and endless crazy letters, and fought my battle with cool calmness, I'm sure he did not always feel.

Thanks to Paddy Summerfield for his advice, understanding, and most of all his empathy.

Thanks to Jeff Rice for his listening skills, and encouragement in writing this book. Also thanks to both Jeff and Lydia for reading the first draft, your kind words made me want to continue.

Thanks to Marie Martin who wrote me such a tender letter, and knew from her own experience, not once but twice, what I was suffering, your words meant so much.

Special thanks also to
Lefkos Greco, Andy Ralston, Graham and Linda, Henry Parker, Trish Wilcox-Jones, Elizabeth Yorkshades, Marie Darkins, Zoe McIntosh, George Cannon, Martin Garner, the real Karen and blonde Karen, Simon Cooper, George and Irena Hrabowy and Dick and Suzann O'Niel. You all in your own ways gave me support, kindness, empathy and sensitivity, it helped so much to know people cared.

A big thanks to everyone who wrote to me or phoned, you all gave me much needed comfort.

ONE IN FOUR

By Joy Ford

Edward Best was my son, he was loved
unconditionally.
When he was stricken with schizophrenia, I wanted
to take him
in my arms and hug away all his fears, as I did
when he was a small boy. But love and hugs
could not protect him any more,
So I dedicate Edwards's story with my love to his
memory,
to all the brave people who battle with mental
illness.
And to Edward's brother, sister, and my husband
who have travelled with me
through the long journey of grief, and trauma
without them I could not have managed.
The poems through out the coming pages were
written by Edward during his illness.
Joy Ford

THE BEGINNING

Scared of rejection
Or to be placed in a fool collection
In a class of my own
Teaching myself to be alone
I try not to listen
But thoughts don't stop,
Making their own conviction
They are causing demolition.
If only I could lock away my brain,
I'm sure I could gain remorse
And find a girl to put me back on course.

We were walking along the side of St. James Park in London on a warm June evening when she turned to me and suddenly said, "Edward's death was his gift to you. You must remember that."

I felt shaken by her words and the familiar hot feeling of unshed tears burned behind my eyes and my throat ached, all I could say was "What?"
"Edward taking his own life, it was his gift to you. You must realise if he had lived he would have killed you or murdered a member of your family."

She spoke with such conviction that my sadness turned in that moment to hot anger; I shook my head wanting to shake her words out of my mind. How dare she I thought, wanting to scream at her so I waited until I could speak calmly.

"Edward was never a violent person," I said at last my voice was shaking "and when he became ill with schizophrenia he remained a gentle person, but he became very fearful of people and situations and tended to keep himself to himself. Before he died he was terrified, he thought people were out to harm him. People with his illness very rarely harm anyone, other than themselves. And that was my greatest fear and I was right to feel like that, because that is what he did, he took his own life. But he did not want to die; he said that continuously the day he made his first attempt. He died on his second attempt that same day, even though we had placed him in a place of safety."

The rest of the evening I felt strained and sad, I found images of my youngest child in the forefront of my mind. My friend, I knew she meant well but like many others she thought "I should be over it by now" just three years after his death, and I'm beginning to realise the death of one's child is not something you "get over" you just learn to live with it. An empty space appeared in my life when my child died and it will remain there forever. Eighteen months after my son's death my mother died, I was sad I grieved and I miss her not being in my life, but I always knew she would one day die, that is the way things are. But I never expected that to happen to my child, I spent time preparing my children to become independent, so they could live happily once I have gone. Nothing prepared me for my child dieing, and with such horrendous injuries, it is the worst pain I have ever experienced, and it does not go away, it sits deep inside me like an icy spot where he once lay and from time to time it rises up and the pain is in my head, my eyes run with tears as I think of him. It's always there on waking I often find myself sighing his name as memory hits me, even before my eyes open.

My friend in her clumsy way was just trying to make me feel better I realised that. But found it hard to forgive her irrational fear of my son, who would never have harmed a soul, even when in a psychotic state. I did not blame her, before Edward became ill I was as ignorant, and thought seriously mentally ill people were to be feared. My only knowledge came from the news papers, T.V. and films were people doing terrible murders and harm are described as 'schizo's' or 'psychos', I knew so little even though I had suffered from bouts of depression most of my adult life, but I have been lucky enough to only require medication and contact with my GP until Edward's death.

Edward lived for two decades, and when I converse with people I still mention him as I do his living older brother and sister, if something arises in a conversation. I will not deny his existence because it may make someone feel uncomfortable. He was part of my life for twenty years, and those years he spent with me helped to make me the person I am today. Edward was my youngest son he died on April 1st 2002, he'd been diagnosed with paranoia schizophrenia ten months before, when a mental health trust started calling me his main carer rather than his mother, and he became a client rather than a young person with a serious illness.

....

Looking back it is difficult to know when the first signs of Edward's illness became apparent. He grew from a loving little boy who was full of curiosity, mischief, laughter, sport loving, and full of non-stop questions, into an introverted teenager, over time the laughter slowly faded, the talking grew less, I thought it was the awkwardness and difficulties of growing up at first, and wasn't worried.

He was a tall lad of six foot by the time he was seventeen. A fine rugby player always in the A team at school, he won a gold medal in the inter-school Judo championships, when he was thirteen, and a bronze medal for skiing around the same time. He was a talented artist, and his art teacher at his prep school became his mentor. I watched his confidence grow as he realised his ability.

He was a good-looking boy, people said he looked like Matt Damon, and certainly in the film "Good Will Hunting" I could see the likeness. He wore baggy clothes his jeans hung around his hips the crutch almost reaching his knees, so to me he looked as if he had a long body and short legs. But it was the fashion and according to him healthy, as he told me "his balls hung free." He loved music, as a small boy he could pick out a tune and play it on the piano by ear, he later learnt to read music as he wanted to learn the saxophone, but his music teacher encouraged him to learn the clarinet first. He loved writing and often scribbled ideas down for a story. He enjoyed his prep school and had many friends and one particular friend, Harry. He hated his next school, this I did not realise until he told me just before he sat his G.C.S.E.'s. It was while at this school he discovered cannabis and started to smoke it regularly from the age of fourteen. Something I feel very strongly helped triggered his illness.

It may help to hear a little about me before I continue with Edwards's story.
I had had a very difficult, miserable and abusive childhood, yet somehow I managed to survive it, but it has left deep problems I still have to cope with, more due to the lack of love and support I felt as a child than anything else. A strong sense of responsibility was impressed on me from the early age of four, just after the birth of my brother, one of my jobs then was to rock him in his pram if he cried, it was a big old 1940's type of pram and I could not reach the handle, it was also highly sprung, and I remember on one occasion becoming very irritated because as soon as I stopped rocking him he started to cry, so I stretched up on tiptoes to reach the top of the handle and gave it a big bounce, and the pram tipped over. My brother cried even more and I was spanked. From then on as the eldest child it was my responsibility to care for my three siblings, when things went wrong it was always my fault. Even now I still feel I am responsible for everything around me.

In my early adulthood I never realised how a pattern can be formed as a child and more often than not you can end up choosing a partner similar to those you have known while growing up. I kind of made that mistake, I had plenty of boy friends but I grew scared if they seemed to become serious, and I'd end the relationship, due to the fact I did not know how to handle anyone seeming to care for me.

Adrian was different and more persistent, he kept me close to him, I lost touch with my own long time friends as I was always with him and his friends, I didn‘t realise what was happening until it was too late. He always had his arm round me, or was holding my hand; I mistook this possessiveness as love. At twenty-one I married him, I believe we did love each other in our own ways. We had both been damaged in our childhoods, and were too young to marry. But once I had there was no going back, for me I thought it would be for my life. A week after we married in 1965 he stood over me as I ironed his shirts, and told me how to do them. I had been ironing shirts for my father and brother since the age of eight, but I was use to being got at, and let him continue criticising the way I ironed, instead of doing what I would do now. Hand him the iron and tell him to do his own bloody ironing. Sadly then I wanted to please, and thought it my responsibility to please the man I married. This feeling was to last for over twenty years.

I'm sure Adrian in his own way loved me, and I was not strong enough then to fight back, maybe if I had things would have been different. There were good times in the beginning, we did things as a family, Adrian like to be in control and manipulated the way he wanted things. I was reasonably happy to let things go and concentrated on bringing up the children. When our first child was born five years after our marriage I had hoped Adrian would start to feel I was a capable person, that did not need watching and criticizing all the time, sadly that did not happen.

I was also very aware that as I had had a difficult childhood, I in turn could continue that circle. But I wanted my children to experience a loving protected childhood and I tried to do the exact opposite to what happened to me. There were faults on both sides I think on reflection I may have been over protective of our children. Adrian's childhood seemed to have been lonely, and from what he has said about his past he missed out on a lot of mothering, though was very spoilt on material things, and as an only child very use to getting his own way, and threw a tantrum if he didn't, a habit he never completely grew out of. I feel my doing things with and for our children caused him to resent what I did, he use to become annoyed at little things I did with them, even when they were older, like helping them fill out a form. He felt as no one ever helped him, or I in doing these things, we should not pass on our knowledge, but let them find out for them selves. I don't know what would have been the correct way; I just followed my instincts and helped when asked.

The years passed and mostly they were happy, mainly because I did not make waves and went along with everything he wanted. We had a daughter in 1969 Jane, a quiet thoughtful and very sensitive child. She had the most wonderful imagination, and lived in a world of calm, love and make- believe, until she started her secondary school. She had a caring nature and loved doing things and making things for those around her. Her gentleness made growing up hard for her; she took so many things to heart, and suffered through other people's careless and thoughtless comments. At secondary school she was badly bullied and this affects her out look on herself to this day. She was also witness to the terrible years Adrian and I suffered at the end of our marriage – whereas Jack and Edward had other places to go to get away from it. She saw and heard it all. Even so she has grown into one of the kindest and most loving of people I have ever known.

In 1971 Jack was born. He too was also a sensitive loving and artistic child, but also a rascal he was into everything. Always on the go with very little fear for anything and in consequence we spent many hours in A&E over the years, due to his daredevil acts. I could not take my eyes of him for a moment, I had to try and be one step ahead of him. He had a shocking temper when a toddler, and thought nothing of throwing himself on the ground screaming, wherever we were if things did not go his way, and he learnt the hard way, that no, meant no by me, how ever much he screamed and yelled. Due to glue ear he was often deaf on and off through out his childhood, he also suffered from dyslexia, this made learning very hard for him. He struggled though out his school years and had tough times, yet he managed to get himself through it, and became a stronger person inconsequence. He has grown into a caring and loving husband and father.

November 1981 Edward was born, he was a combination of both his sister and brother, having the dare devil character of Jack and the self-awareness and lone interests of Jane, he was also the brightest of the three children and learnt quickly. He spent his childhood years trying to catch up with his older brother and sister. Both the older two were wonderful to Edward. They were always there for him, and delighted in all his achievements, he was a very much-loved addition to our family.

Two years after Edward's birth the cracks in our marriage had become wide gaps. Jack always refers to it "as the time dad changed," Adrian had always been a controller and manipulator but around this time these things became very much more pronounced. Around this time return trains from London where he worked were often delayed, and he would return from work late. Strangely when the trains started to run on time again some months later, he slipped into a very deep depression. He'd sit for hours out in the garden just staring ahead. I tried to find out what was wrong, and tried to encourage him to talk, but he would just become very angry with me. I have my own thoughts on this matter, but they are only thoughts. He had always been a bit of a Victorian father, but after this episode he distanced himself from his children even more especially the older two. Adrian was also a perfectionist and loved perfect things around him, I was ageing and growing plumper, and was not the same person he married. I had gained a lot of self-confidence and myself esteem had improved with age so I started to fight back. This sadly ended in the break down of our marriage. Adrian found the change in me hard to cope with, he'd become too use to me being the quiet little doormat, but I had found my courage and could not go back. I felt I had the right to say, think and do what I wanted to do, not all the time, but he could not compromise. I felt awful and very guilty ending the marriage, and hated what I was doing to those I cared about, including Adrian. But in the situation I was in then I would either have driven a knife through him or myself, which was how bad I felt. In the last few years of our marriage I became afraid of him because the stronger I grew the more nasty he became towards me.

Edward was fourteen when his father and I were going through a very difficult divorce. That was obviously hard on all three of the children, and even more so for Edward who was coping with adolescent crises as well. I took out a loan the year he was fifteen and took him to Florida for two weeks. We went with his friend Harry and his mother, she was going through a difficult time too, and we both felt the boys needed a break from the family stress. I'm so glad I did that it was one of the very best holidays I had with Edward, and the last time I was to see him trouble free, young, and really happy. The memories and photos of that holiday have become very precious.

As I said my marriage had been floundering for sometime, when Edward was thirteen he said to me "Excuse me mum but why don't you divorce dad?" I apologised to him for all the arguing, and he said, "That's what I've heard all my life, but it's getting worse."

He was right it was, I could never do or say anything right any more, and lived in fear of my then husband, life was very stressful, with constant rows, when ever we were together. Adrian seemed to have some kind of demon inside him, which could not stop going on at me, until he had expelled all his hate and frustration. I tried several ways to deal with it, from trying to talk to him to find out what was wrong, but he seemed to think I had a problem, so I tried ignoring him and continuing as normal, but he would goad me until I snapped. I tried to reply calmly and quietly treating the monologue of words as normal, while inside I felt sicker and sicker, tried fighting back, but nothing was right. I often use to end up crouched into a foetal position with my fingers in my ears sobbing as I tried to shut him out. I'd be crying and pleading with him to stop, but he seemed unable to, and this constant talking at me in a monosyllable tone would go on often into the small hours, non stop his voice filling my whole head, I didn't know how to stop him.

In desperation I spoke to our GP about it, he suggested I tried moving myself from the situation. I then would walk out when he started and walk for a couple of hours whatever the time of day or the weather, sometimes I find a dark corner on the common and cry. Always when I returned he was waiting for me and would continue on at me as if I had not been away for a couple of hours. Sometimes I begged him to just hit me and get it over with, anything to stop the continuous drone of his voice. I still even now have a terrible fear of ever saying anything that may be adverse, in case someone treats me that way again. It makes things difficult in all relationships because I never say what's bothering me; I shut it up inside myself. Physical cruelty is bad enough but mental cruelty is beyond words, and no one can ever see the damage, it's not like a black eye or a broken limb, it's in the mind where no one knows. Some years later my GP looked through my notes and said "Joy this problem has been going on for over ten years. I think it is your husband that has the problem, not you, he needs to come and see me." He suggested I tried relate, and to persuade Adrian to pay him a visit. That proved impossible, though I did go to

Relate.

Living that way with Adrian was no way for any one to live, and certainly not something I wanted my three children to witness. It was stressful enough for me so what it did to Edward and his sister and brother I dread to think. I also felt Adrian must have been as unhappy, why else would he behave in this way, he could not have been happy living with me. He kept saying he was trying to consol me, but I never needed consoling until he started on at me. He claimed he behaved the way he did because he loved me and I would say, “If this is love, I’ll do without it.” It was a vicious circle, certainly our three children were stressed and suffering by the atmosphere at home. I tried going to relate in 1994 and when Adrian was invited to attend by letter he refused to go. He claimed sometime later that he thought I was attending Relate to learn how to relate to people as he thought I had a problem. Even though he drove me to Oxford to attend, and he sat out side by a notice that said “Relate formally known as Marriage Guidance.” In November 1995 I saw a solicitor who wrote to explain how unhappy I was by the situation we found our selves in, and explained I wanted the two of us to seek help and to sort things out, again this was ignored, and he threw the letter away.

After a terrible Christmas and miserable winter I filed for a divorce at the end of February 1996. Then Adrian began to see how serious things were between us, and started to plead with me to stop the divorce. He kept telling me he was now being kind to me, and could not understand my saying “You shouldn‘t have to tell someone you’re being kind.” He promised he would not treat me the way he had been, part of me wanted to believe him and call the divorce off. I was scared at what I was doing and I had no idea if I could cope or what the future held. But I could not go back as all my trust for Adrian had gone, I couldn’t believe he would change sadly when my trust went so did my love.

My thirty odd years of marriage ended on the seventh of January 1997. Though Adrian still remained living with me, and wanting meals and washing done it took a court order for him too leave on March 13th 1997, the house was sold in the August of that year, and I and the children moved to a smaller place in the same village.
From that day I started to make a life for myself and my three children, all three were still living at home.

Though money was very tight with a mortgage to pay, all the other household expenses and a fifteen year old to support on one low salary, I was a far more relaxed and happier person, and this reflected on the atmosphere of the home, and those living with me. I also did not need anti-depressants any more, even though I was constantly harassed by Adrian for the next few years. The constant depressed state I had been living in lifted, and I felt happy and at ease. I still had several run-ins with

Adrian, he use to tell Edward he was going to end his life and Ed' would return very stressed, and once in tears. I tried suggesting that Ed' did not see his father for a while, but he was beginning to feel responsible for his fathers happiness. I tried talking to Adrian, but he never listened, he was too busy trying to say his part.

Adrian had had his own business then and that became part of his marriage settlement, I wanted nothing from him, all I asked for was enough for a deposit on a house so the children and I had somewhere to go. I left the dividing of everything to the courts. Adrian had a choice from the council of three different apartments, he told Edward he had chosen the apartment that had only one room and was rather small, because when I saw it I'd feel sorry for him and ask him to move back in with me. Edward also told me to stop writing to Adrian as he underlined certain words in red and made them into sentences that read something different to what I had written. I only wrote to try to get him to understand why I had had to end our relationship, as he harassed me constantly. But I was far stronger now and all his methods failed, but I do feel he used Edward at times to get at me.

Edward did really well in his GCSE's passing all eight with mostly B and C grades and achieving an A. Star in Art. At that time he was very excited at his results and had plans of going onto art college he wanted to study animation, after he took his A-levels at sixth form college, he was still then reasonably out going and in contact with his friends. He went clubbing and also attended raves, Reading music festival, and was into Rap Music. I'm sure he experimented with drugs, but apart from nicotine I do not believe he was addicted to any, but I believe cannabis played a big part in his illness. He lived at home apart from the year of 2000, when he moved to London for a time, but returned home regularly, that was the only year when I did not know where he was or what he was doing. I think then he was beginning to become aware that his mental state was not as it should be. I believe he moved away hoping a changed environment would help him turn his life around.

His happiness and ambition did not last. At the end of his sixteenth year Edward had given up sport, some of that was due to injuries especially to his right ankle and knee, he was out of rugby for one whole season. It was around this time his motivation had begun to fade. He saw less and less of his friends, kept claiming he'd fallen out with them or did not like them any more. He dropped out of sixth-form college twice, but found it very difficult to look for work or find anything to do of interest. He seemed to spend more time sleeping in the day and staying awake at night.

In his seventeenth year I worried about him constantly, I feared he was involved with drugs and looked for signs. I read everything I could on drugs and teenage culture. I challenged him endlessly and he would become angry with me, and I felt guilty for not trusting him, but I still sensed something was not right. We had many long discussions, at times quite heated, on drugs and their affects on a person. I realised he was more enlightened than I on the subject.

At the time there was a lot from the media and their involvement in cannabis and the down grading of the drug, with the government and some medical people almost giving the thumbs up that is was a safe drug. At this time you could not open a newspaper, put on the radio or TV without hearing about how harmless cannabis was.

Edward started to join the marches in London and we had some strong arguments about smoking cannabis. At nearly eighteen he thought he knew it all, and had the back up of the media to support his argument, I was just his mum what did I know.
It was around this time he told me he'd been smoking cannabis on and off from the age of fourteen and I was horrified. I caught him once smoking it in his bedroom, and forbade him to ever use it in our home. I actually threatened to call the police if he ever did it again, though I doubt that I would have if it had happened again. The one thing I will say about Edward even when really seriously mentally ill, he always showed me love and respect.

I have to admit at the time I was confused about cannabis, there was so much coming from the media, even saying it was safer than alcohol, I wasn't sure what to believe. At the end of April 1997 I had become friends with a man who had been recently widowed, his wife of nearly twenty-five years died in November 1996. I became Nick's support as he journeyed through his grief, I held him when he wept, and listened when he talked, I had lost a sister in June of 96 so could empathise with what he was going through, sometimes we cried together over our lost loved ones. He too believed cannabis was a soft drug, and understood Edward smoking it, more than I did. He and Edward became pretty good friends their common interest in music being a bond. But I decided to be cautious where my son was concerned, as I did not know enough about the drug. He still continued to smoke it when he went out.

Often he went to clubs and pubs by himself during this time, not meeting up with anyone this worried me, but he always claimed he was cool and not to worry. He wasn't earning money and neither could I afford to give him any, apart from when his father gave him money he did not have any, so his smoking of cannabis was very spasmodic as were his outings. I had by then started to recognise the changes in him when he had been smoking cannabis, he was far less receptive, with no motivation at all, and a little paranoid.

Over time the paranoia increased, he accused me of stalking him, searching his room and belongings. He'd wake at night really believing someone had been in his room while he was asleep, he often cried out in his sleep. He started to put things against his bedroom door so it was difficult to open. He couldn't have a bath or a shower unless he cleaned the bath first, even if it had already just been cleaned. He had to have a clean towel every time he washed, and inspected eating utensil before he would eat. He became a vegetarian for several months. Then changed from being really clean to not washing or changing his clothes, I would nag him and his brother use to tell him he stank, but at that time he knew better than any one. He would boast that he had too much confidence and I would tell him I didn't think he had any confidence or self-esteem, but that he covered up with arrogance.

At times he would not speak for days, just teenage grunts, and spent most of his time in his room. Then at other times he was very receptive and quite talkative. On one of these occasions he told me he thought he was suffering from schizophrenia, I asked him why he thought that, he just said, "I don't know but I think I am." I told him he had to have a reason to believe that, and if I arranged for him to see a doctor, then they would also want to know why he thought he had schizophrenia. He said he had looked it up on the inter-net and had he several symptoms. Yet when asked he could not tell me one symptom.

Over the past few days he had self diagnosed several ailments in himself, both physical and mental. The day before he thought he was suffering from claustrophobia. I will never forgive myself for ignoring this conversation and treating it as "another of Edward's imaginings." Now I realise he was very aware there was something wrong and was searching for an answer. I wish I had just taken him to the doctor on the day he felt he was suffering from schizophrenia.

At that time I knew very little about mental illness as such and even less about schizophrenia and psychosis, all I had to go on was the media image of someone to be feared. A person who had a split personality; one half being a cold-blooded murder, the other gentle and charming.

My son was not a person to fear neither did he have a split personality. I wish I had found out about the illness at that time, but then I had no idea how to start, I did not have a computer the ones Edward used was his fathers, or his brothers. I could find information on Cancer, forms of dementia, Parkinson's, M.E. or M.S. endless ailments I could have found leaflets readily available in doctors surgeries, libraries, etc. But information on mental illness was kept in the dark.

At another of these receptive times he told me he had left sixth- form college because he had been gang raped after his drink had been spiked. At the time I had no reason to disbelieve him, the way he said it happened sounded very plausible and I was really shocked, he begged me not to tell any one, and he said I did not know the people involved. He didn't want the police or college to know, so I was relieved that he felt able to talk to me. He did not want anyone in the family to know, but did not mind my talking to Nick. I hugged him and suggested he went for an aids test, and that he should visit our GP

Nick and I took Edward to Oxford for his Aids test- the result was negative. I also went with him to visit our GP he was away and we saw someone else. I explained how Edward was behaving and how worried I was about him, and then I left Edward with the GP so they could talk in private. When he came out he said the doctor had told him he was suffering with depression, but did not think he needed any medication. I brought him some St. Johns Wart the in thing at that time for depression. I realise now the gang rape possibly did not happen that it was probably one of his first psychotic experiences if not the first. Now I will never know the truth of it all.

Just after his eighteenth Birthday in November 1999, Edward suddenly announced that he was moving to London, that Reading and Oxford held nothing for him. I was totally shocked and very upset I did not want him to go; neither did the rest of the family or friends I spoke to. But I was afraid of going against him in fear of making him more determined. One friend suggested I forbid him to go, but he was over eighteen and I believed he would have just left home and gone to London, and I would not hear from him again.

Nick was still in my life and our friendship by now had turned into love and in September 1999 we had started to think about finding a place so we could live together. My three children had accepted him and were pleased I was happy. Edward at that time seemed really happy about us making a home together. He even sat with us when we had found two houses we liked but could not decide on which village we wanted to live in. He said to us both where do you see yourself living when you are seventy. We both said Blewbury and the problem was solved. Edward liked the house though it only had two bedrooms. Edwards room would have to be used for guest on rare occasions, but he was happy to sleep downstairs when this happened. He asked if he could also have the use of a small room downstairs to play his music and entertain his friends, to which we agreed. He already knew some people in Blewbury and seemed to be looking forward to moving as much as Nick and I were. We'd checked on buses to college because he wanted to return to take his A-levels, and at that moment in time, I really believed he had turned the corner, and was at last beginning to grow up, he seemed well and happy.

So the sudden wanting to move to London seemed really out of place, I offered to stay where I was living and not move in with Nick. I thought maybe he didn't want things to change and I was prepared to put everything on hold. But he convinced me that it was not a problem for him, that he liked Nick and thought it was a good idea. He said he was going to

London, wherever I chose to live and nothing was going to stop him. I offered him a flat on his own locally and driving lessons, I tried everything to try a persuade him to stay near his family. But when I discovered him looking on the Internet for hostels in London I gave in. A flat was found for him I paid three months rent in advance as well as the bond. I also put another three thousand pounds in a bank account for him as an emergency fund. I only had this money, because I had just sold my house and after paying my half for the Blewbury house there was money left over. Edward promised to go to the youth employment centre and sign on as soon as he arrived, and check out Camberwell college to find out what A levels he required to attend that college to study Art, and see where he could take his A levels, he refused any help from me in looking for these places, saying he wasn‘t a child and I was not responsible for him anymore.

In January 2000 he moved to Balham. His father took him and all his clothes, bedding and utensils I had brought for his new life in Balham, the rest of his things I put into the attic of my new home in Blewbury where I had just moved to, they are still there to this day.

I phoned him regularly and at first he seemed very happy though I worried all the time. We travelled up to London to see him one Saturday morning, after speaking to him the evening before and saying we would like to visit him. He asked if I had a spare plant for his flat and we put one in the car that

Saturday morning. Nick, Ed's sister Jane and I arrived at his flat at lunch time, after an hour and half journey in very heavy traffic, he was not in. We walked down to the shops near by, thinking maybe he'd gone shopping for some lunch. I had had this vision of him entertaining his friends and leading a normal student life. I know that was how he envisaged his life in London, and I desperately wanted him to find happiness. We hung around his flat for an hour and a half; I tried phoning his mobile and could hear it ring inside the flat. In the end feeling angry I left him a note and the plant and we went home.

Late that evening I managed to get him on the phone; he seemed very detached and unconcerned about our journey and waiting for him. He claimed he been out with friends he'd met the night before. I'd had the feeling he was inside his flat when we were there, but didn't want to come to the door. He never went anywhere without his mobile phone and I'd heard that ringing inside the flat.

He use to come home most weekends, at times we'd get a phone call late at night to say "Mum I'm at the train station can you come and get me." Though this use to annoy Nick he always went and collected him, but the fact that Edward claimed he wanted to be treated like an adult, but could not take the responsibility of getting himself from the station to Blewbury, did at times put a strain on my relationship with Nick.

He'd phone about bills and TV license and though I would advise him in the same way as I had his sister, when she had first started to live away from home. He could never sort anything out and I found myself doing it all for him. I also found that he never went near a college or a job centre, that he spent most of his time in his flat, and had found a place that he could phone for food etc and have it delivered. The money I had put into a bank account for emergencies was being used to pay for this. I tried to explain that I could not help him out once that money had gone, and he would have to start taking care of himself, and in April he would have to start paying rent.

It was then that I heard for the first time something I was going to continuously hear for the rest of Edwards's short life.

"Don't worry mum, I'm going to get a job in McDonald's, and work in a pub in the evenings, and get my A levels and then go onto Art College." I believe he really did want to do this, that he believed he could do it as well, but he was completely unable to motivate himself, he just had no energy or the confidence. I never realised at this time just how unwell he was. I was aware something was wrong with my youngest child, and that he was still very dependent on me, but I had no understanding as to what the problem was. There were plenty of people telling me what to do and how I should treat him; most advice was for me to be really hard on him and cut him out of my life, let him fend for himself completely. There were times when I felt really angry with him and in complete despair, but somewhere at the back of my mind I had this feeling there was something terribly wrong and I could not let him go, because he needed me. He behaved like a child of fourteen or fifteen; he seemed to me, to be stuck emotionally in that age, unable to move on.

He came home one weekend in early March with a terrible black eye, he said he had done it roller blading, I never found out how he did it. A couple of weekends after that he told me he had to go to court for being in a fight, that out of the six of them in the fight he was the only one to be arrested. The story he told did not ring true, but no matter how much I questioned him he would not tell me what was really wrong. It was over two years later that I discovered he had stolen traveller's cheques off an American he had met in a pub.

Then I discovered he had left his flat and was back in Oxfordshire living with his father. The two weeks before that he had stayed in a bed sit in Paddington where the toilets were so dirty, that he used to go to Paddington Station for the use of a toilet and to wash. I never found out why he had left his flat in Balham with a month's rent still paid for. I did discover that all the money I had put into the bank for him was gone, and that he had nothing left, and his last two weeks in London he was destitute. All I can imagine is that he had some sort of delusion concerning his Balham flat, and felt he could not return. Several times I wrote to him during his stay in London pleading with him to trust me and tell me what was troubling him, I explained how much I loved him and that he was my son and I wanted to help him, that I would never judge him, I just wanted to help him, that I was there for him what ever the problem. He always came home after one of my letters and I hoped he would talk but he never did.

He was given a date for his court case in Hammersmith, and I said I would go with him. He became very angry and insisted he did not want me there, and I had no need to worry. We had a few arguments on this subject but he was quite adamant he did not want me to be in court to support him. Just before the court case he went to meet a girl he found through a chat room, they had been communicating for some time before they arrange to meet. He was really very excited and very happy; he was convinced he already loved her.

She came from Kent and it was quite a journey for them to meet up, they met up several times in London before he brought her home to stay one weekend. She was a lovely girl, tall, willowy, and beautiful the same age as Edward, but far more mature. She was friendly and out going and I thought things may improve, as she was sensible and started to encourage Edward to return to college and to sign on and start looking for work. As Edward was so strongly against me going to court with him, Katy offered to accompany him I realised he had probably told her the true story, and I was grateful for her offer. He at least had one friendly face with him.

On his return from court he told me he'd been put on two years probation and had a fine of nine hundred pounds, plus community work for a year. I knew that whatever he had been in court for it was not just a fight. I had no idea how he was ever going to pay the nine hundred pounds; it seemed to be just another problem that had to be dealt with. He started his community work in the local Oxfam Shop, which he seemed to enjoy apart from the having to get up early. He brought odd gifts home for me and seemed to be settling down. The council had given him a bond so he could find a flat locally. He was still seeing Katy and was very happy for a short while, something I had not seen for a long time.

Then because of the logistics of Katy living in Kent and him in Oxfordshire, the call of London took hold of Edward again. He was determined he was going back to London and started to pack his bags. The very last of my savings went on a flat in Camberwell, but only two months in advance; this was in late August 2000. I also went with him to the local job centre and the council where I introduced him and explained he was moving into the area. He was told to call in and see the people as soon as he moved in and they could register him. His Probation Officer was changed to one in the area he was moving to. I again brought him new bedding and other things for his flat, plus a fridge. I don't know what happened to the things brought for his other flat; I imagine they were with his father. I explained that I could do no more to help him financially and that he really did have to look for work, and do his A- levels at night school so he could attend Camberwell Art College, something he insisted he really wanted to do. I had hoped with his friendship with Katy his life would start to really work out.

The happiness lasted about a month, then the old paranoia started up again, he thought Katy was seeing someone else. He came home for a weekend really upset, because she was working in the Co-Op and had told him she had to work until ten, one evening. He didn't believe her and thought she was meeting another young man. I told him our local Co-Op was open until ten, so she was more than likely telling him the truth. We talked about trust that weekend, and I explained how important that was in a relationship and that if he really loved Katy he should trust her, as she had given him no real reason to doubt her. At that time he seemed to agree and returned to London in a better frame of mind. Sadly it did not last he returned another weekend to say they had broken up.

He was really upset, he said he had been abusive to her because she had worked late and helped out at a local village fete, before she had called on him. He said she was very tired and he had been drinking and he wanted to have sex, but she wanted to rest. That he became angry with her and kept on and on at her for keeping him waiting he had reduced her to tears and she had walked out. He felt bad about the way he had behaved towards her and even worse at making her cry. I suggested he phoned her and explained how sorry he was for hurting her and explain why, but I also told him it did not mean that she would want to see him again as she might not, but at least that would clear the air and hopefully they could remain friends. He didn't phone her and when ever I brought the subject up he would say "Oh this is just some game we play, Katy is always playing games with me, she understands, I don't need to phone her."

Edward's mood became lower over the next few weeks, he became increasingly depressed, I tried to encourage him to see a doctor, but he refused. I phoned his probation officer and explained how worried I was about Edward. She said she had noticed a change in him, though he always kept his appointment, on some visits he would not speak at all, and then on others he was quite chatty but seemed very unhappy.

Then one evening early in October 2000 I had a phone call from the police in Camberwell, they had taken Edward into custody, due to the fact that he had been standing outside his flat shouting abuse at people standing at a bus stop. They said he was very drunk and that he had had a bread knife in his jeans pocket. They told me not to worry and not to travel to London, as he was too drunk. They were waiting for the police doctor to visit him and that they did not know if they were going to charge him at that moment.

Edward came home the following day and I knew something was dreadfully wrong. He claimed the police had fitted him up, that they had broken into his flat and put red paint all over his cloths making it look like blood. That they were coming to get him. He did have some sort of red ink on his sweatshirt he was wearing; I tried to explain to him that forensics could prove it was not blood. But he claimed I didn't understand he seemed very scared. He also complained about people on the train while he travelled to Oxfordshire he said they were weird, that they stared at him, and some were making comments about his baseball cap. That he had to talk to one man who was very well dressed in a suit and tie for laughing at his cap, that he would not have expected some one like that to behave so rudely. He did not stay long he seemed very restless and wanted to return to London. Edward was taken to court for this episode for being drunk and carrying a weapon, another six months was added to his probation. I now believe it was another delusional episode. I phoned his probation officer the following day and told her how Edward had behaved and that I was very concerned about his mental health. She said she would try and get an assessment for him.

While in London this time Edward had met up with an old school friend, and just after this episode he stayed with Edward after a quarrel with his mother. At first it seem to work out then one weekend late in October Edward came home and said he had asked Jim to be out of the flat by the time he returned home. I asked him why and he said that Jim and some of his friends had soaked a lot of cigarettes in water to get all the nicotine out and they had tried to inject it into him. I didn't know what to say to this or how to handle the situation, Nick just felt he was having me on and that I was a fool to listen to him. I could understand Nick's reaction, the most he had ever seen of Edward he was causing problems for me to solve, apart from when Nick and I had first met, at that time Nick was suffering himself and not really aware of what Edward was like then.

So now to Nick it appeared to be my son taking advantage of me all the time. But I knew the real person, the Edward who had been so very self aware for one so young, and sensitive to other people, some where deep down that loving caring person was still there. These irrational thoughts and behaviour had to have an explanation. I again spoke to his probation officer and the mental health assessment date was given. I don't know what I hoped from this assessment, but something more than. "Yes there is a mental problem, and he will needed treatment sometime in the future," and that was it, things were just left. I wondered why there was such a thing as an assessment, as all it did was confirm my fears about Edward's mental health. There was no help for my son or any advice as what to do next, just nothing.

On the weekend near to November the eighth Edward came home for his nineteenth Birthday, I made a special meal and asked family to join us. Edward was so down, I'd never seen him like this, and he was also slightly hostile and spoke quite sharply to people. He opened his presents but did not seem particularly pleased with any of them. At the meal he kept his head down and did not speak, it was an excruciating meal and I think everyone was pleased when it was over. When Edward's brother and fiancée were ready to leave Edward asked them for a lift to the station, he was returning to London, and not staying over as I had hoped he would.
I rang him the following evening, and every evening that week, and some days I even rang from work, but I could never get hold of him and I was worried sick. On the Friday evening I rang his father and had made up my mind if he had not heard from him I would travel to London the following day. On ringing his father I discovered Edward was there and had been for several days. Edward had phoned his father earlier in the week to say that the flat had been broken into, and his things had been set on fire. I found out later that Edward had burnt all of his own things and those he could not burn he had destroyed. The only thing that he had failed to destroy was his fridge, that after he had done this he had asked his father to collect him, and he was now living there.

He came to visit me about a week later his story of the break in seemed genuine and I felt really sorry for him, he'd not only lost all his clothes and C.D. collection and other personal things, plus his birthday presents, but his art portfolio and that could not be replaced. He said he wanted to go back to London, he had been doing his community work with a removal firm and he wanted to continue with them. I was not happy about this and said no and that I could not afford to pay for any more flats or bail him out of his debts as I had been doing. A half sister who lived in Hertford offered him a place to stay; it was only twenty minutes to London from their home. I explained the difficulties that Edward was having and at nineteen he'd never worked neither had he continued his education. They were good caring people and still were willing for him to stay. I felt that he would be safer living with them and they would be able to monitor his mental health and would also be aware if he was messing with drugs, something I was never sure about. Steve my sister's husband had knowledge of drugs and was involved in helping people who had drug problems. Edward accepted their offer and once again I waved him off to London. I think they had a difficult time with Edward, though to this day I don't know the full story of what went on, I think they want to spare my feelings. I do believe Edward was very ill but none of us realised. I'm really grateful to them for caring for Edward over those few weeks; at least he had been in a safe environment just before he completely broke down.

The last weekend of November Edward rang to say he was coming home next weekend, I explained that Nick and I would not be there as I was visiting my brother and his family in Cromer. Edward still came and stayed with his father, when I returned on the Sunday evening Edwards father rang to ask if Edward was with me. I explained that I had only just returned and had not seen him. Then I was told when Edward arrived on the Saturday he had been very loving, and tactile something he had not been for sometime. He told his father how much he loved him and how pleased he was to see him. In the afternoon he went out to watch the local football team play, on his return he told his father they had won because he had used the power of his mind. That he was going to use the power of his mind to help them get through to the cup final and win the cup. That evening he fell out with his father and walked out.

This was the year 2000, when it rained continuously all through autumn and winter, and that Saturday night was no exception. Edward went out in the pouring rain with no coat or money, and rang his father at four thirty in the morning. He was picked up in Didcot over ten miles from where his father lived, just four miles from where I lived. He was covered in mud and soaked right through, and totally exhausted; his father bathed him and put him to bed. When asked later where he had been, he explained he had walked through fields and met three ghosts who had really scared him. But when he had raised his arms and said, "Go from this place" they had disappeared. On the Sunday they were to have lunch at his grandmothers, someone Edward had always got on well with. But at the door he suddenly refused to go in and asked to be taken to the local railway station. His request was refused and he walked off and no one knew where he was. Steve and my sister Lucy who had also been visiting friends in the area had to return to Hertford without him. I spent a sleepless night worrying, I did not realise this was to become the first of many.

The following lunchtime with still no word from Edward I went to the local police station, it had been twenty-four hours since he had walked off and I reported him missing. I also explained that he was behaving very irrationally and I was really worried about his mental health. The police were understanding asked for a recent photo, and due to his mental state took my concern seriously. At about seven thirty Tuesday evening Steve phoned, to say the police had found Edward in Stevenage and that he had been put into Steve and Lucy's care. The following evening Steve phoned to say they were bringing Edward home and that he needed a doctor urgently. That he had been awake all night talking and moving about but they were unable to communicate with him. I phoned Edward's old GP who had known him since a baby, and after explaining the situation he agreed to see him, even though he was not his patient any more. Then Edward refused to leave Lucy and Steve's home, Lucy rang me from a neighbour, as she was afraid Edward would hear her talking to me. I told her to phone the police and explain things to them, that I gave her permission to do that, and not to feel bad about it. That was the only thing I could think of, I knew my son was desperately ill, even though I did not know what was wrong, I was worried not only about Edward but Lucy and Steve's safety as well.

After talking to Lucy the phone rang again this time it was Edward, he sounded very agitated and complained to me that Steve was trying to make him sit down and he did not want to and for me to tell Steve that, and that he would not come and see me until Friday, he spoke in short sharp sentences and sounded nothing like my son. I told him that was fine I would see him on Friday. I then asked Edward to let me speak to Steve. When he came on the phone I asked him to leave Edward, suggested he just let him be, unless he looked as if he might damage himself or either of them, and to wait for the police. If he wanted to walk about and keep talking, to let him do that.

They phoned me after the police had been to say they had taken him to the Queen Elizabeth Hospital in Welling Garden City. It seemed the police were surprised by his reaction to them, he had sat calmly and explained he could not leave the house because he was the son of God and was in touch with the Pope that their minds were working on collecting all the Evil in the world and destroying it. That he could not leave until he had completed the task. When the police explained that they thought he should see a doctor. He said, "If you the police think I should see a doctor I will." He stood ready to walk out with them. They had not expected him to be so co-operative towards them, but that was Edward all the way through his illness, always respectful to those in authority, this I feel was part of his downfall. If he had appeared more aggressive towards doctors and such like, his illness would have been taken far more seriously. I sure the Fair Mile would not have ignored him and aloud him to walk to his death, if he had acted more aggressively. The one thing that really saddens me is the fact that the police handcuffed him, after he left sisters flat.

The following poem was written for Katy,

KATY

It's kind of hard with you not around.
In my heart is where I keep a friend.
Memories give me strength I need to proceed.
The strength I need to believe.
Hard thoughts, big, I just can't let die.
Wish I could turn back the hand of time.
Still can't believe you're gone
I'd give anything to hear half your breath.
I know your living somewhere else
It's kind of hard with you not around.

THE ILLNESS

I'm twisted up in the mind
It's a crooked world.
I'm burning up inside
It's a crooked world
My hearts on a beat
Down to my feet.
Feeling it's coming up
Coming up from concrete.
I'm twisted up in the mind

SECTION 28

After a sleepless night I left home early without breakfast and caught a rush hour train to Paddington and started my journey to Hertfordshire and the Queen Elizabeth Hospital. Due to flooding on many train lines, it took me seven and a half hours to reach the hospital, I was so worried about my son I didn't stop for a break, and only had a small bottle of water during the travel. It was almost dark by the time I reached the hospital. The psychiatric ward was on the top floor it was a locked ward. I found Edward in a tiny room the door closed with a window in it so a nurse who continually walked past could see the patient. The room was white and clinical, the walls bare apart from a paper with a cross drawn on it by Edward, stuck on the wall at the head of his bed. His father Adrian was already there he was sitting on the only chair, and Edward was sitting at the foot of the bed. Neither were speaking when I arrived, as I walked in Edward burst into tears, and I put my arms around him, trying not to cry myself. We stayed huddled together for some time, he sobbed "Why am I here mum, I haven't done anything wrong. I just love God, what's wrong with that."

I sat on the bed beside him and agreed that loving God was fine, and I tried to explain that he had not done anything wrong. I told him he was in hospital, because we were concerned about him and that he was very ill. He was really unable to grasp any of this, he did not think he was ill, and was convinced he was in some kind of prison. He thought it was some sort of government plot and the people in the ward were there for political brain washing. He saw the doctors and nurses as being against him and trying to harm him. He thought the food was poisoned and wouldn't eat anything, and showed us tablets he had not taken, though the staff thought he had. He told us he was the Son of God and he explained he was here to help make the world become a better place. In a bedside drawer he had found a tattered bible and he sat on the windowsill of this sparse little room, that had bars at the window and read his father and I extracts from the bible. In between the readings he'd stop and explain his interpretations of his readings. Always when I think of this, I see it as the "Sermon on the window sill". While he read I ate a beetroot sandwich, Adrian had given to me, the first thing I had eaten all day, and it tasted wonderful.

On my arrival on the ward I had been told that a

doctor would want to talk to us at sometime, and while we waited with Edward after he had tired of the bible reading, he asked if we would take him to buy a sandwich, a drink, and a bible. We agreed to the sandwich and drink, but I explained it might not be possible to buy a bible as it was late and the shops were closing. We made our way to the main door and an alarm went off, making us jump. A nurse joined us and said Edward could not leave the ward. We explained we would not leave the hospital, but just go to the canteen for refreshments, if he could come with us and we would take care of him. They refused and Edward was escorted back to his room. Then they deactivated the main door so Adrian and I could leave the ward.

As I had thought it was not possible to buy a bible, there were only a few shops local to the area, most were closed, but we found a Spar and brought the food Edward had requested, and I also brought some wash things as I noticed Edward did not seem to have any of his own.

On our return we went back into the little room, Edward seemed excited and made a grab for the shopping bag. He searched through it and then tipped everything onto the bed. "Where's the bible?" he demanded of me. I explained the situation. But he wasn't listening, he was angry; he accused me of not buying one on purpose. He said I didn't want him to have one, I'm afraid at this point I burst into tears, I felt at a complete loss, I didn't know how to deal with this person, he was so unlike the Edward I knew. I was exhausted by the journey, had hardly eaten anything all day, and had drunk only a small bottle of water since leaving home, and I was worried sick about my son. I'd never seen any one psychotic before, and the fact it was my youngest child in this state was very frightening. Here I was his mother and I felt completely helpless, and now he was raving at me and thinking I was against him for not buying him a bible. He was too ill to even understand why I was crying. I managed to pull myself together, though inside I felt a complete mess, Edward was still not very friendly towards me when Adrian and I were summoned to a meeting. He was also very annoyed that he could not attend the meeting, and felt his father and I were now included in the plot against him.

The nurse showed us to into a large room around a long table sat an array of people, some in white coats. The man at the top of the table introduced himself, he was the consultant physiatrist, and then the rest of the people introduced themselves and explained what they did. I don't know if Adrian took it all in, but I certainly didn't, there were art therapists, drama therapists, assistants, students, nurses, doctors, it was completely over whelming.

We sat by the consultant and he explained that he could not stress how very ill Edward was, and that he was hovering on the edge of schizophrenia. He said we must get him onto medication straight away to stop that happening. I can remember saying "Do what ever is needed to help him, please do it as soon as possible." Adrian felt exactly the same; we did not see any point in delaying things. Then came the statement, "But he does not live in this area, we will have to transfer him back to Oxfordshire for treatment, where he originally came from, we need an address to put on our records, and do you know the name of any mental hospitals in your area."

I gave him the Blewbury address, and also the name of three hospitals, that I knew of. It took a week to transfer Edward on the twelfth of December 2000 he arrived at the Warnford Hospital in Hedington Oxford. Here I learnt that Blewbury was on the cusp of two county's Oxfordshire and Berkshire, a problem that interfered even more towards the care Edward was to receive.

He was admitted onto Wintle Ward a ward for acute mentally sick people. He was in a room by himself and for the first twenty-four hours he was on continua's watch, and then on a fifteen minute as they assessed him. He was on section 28 of the mental health act while he was assessed. Nick, I, and his father spent hours with the nurses as they took down the history of Edwards's life, and the sort of person he was, when we had noticed any odd behaviour. This was not recorded neither were notes taken at the time of talking. The record of what we said was written in his notes from memory after we had left. This file followed Edward, and after his death when the Berkshire Mental Health Trust were investigated, and a document was made about his care, they used these notes for his history, there were many inaccuracies and when we asked for things to be changed, they refused, once written it seems that‘s what remains mistakes as well.

The hospital was set in pleasant grounds with not enough parking spaces for visitors. The ward Edward was on was an acute ward on the ground floor at first he had a room of his own, and someone for the first twenty four hours sat out side his room, with the door open. It was a mixed ward with mostly older more mature patients; Edward was probably the youngest person there.

There was a dinning room with a pool table in it as well as two long tables and chairs. A sitting room with armchairs and a television. A small kitchen where you could make toast, tea, or coffee, and the smoking room, which was tiny, with seats all around the walls, with book shelves full of books above the chairs. Here most of the people gathered during the day- even the non -smokers if they felt in need of company. It was a clean looked after ward, with attempts to make it look nice. Though when Edward was moved to a dormitory for four, the guy opposite him had very smelly feet, which we all found hard to cope with, and it became a thing to joke about as Edward started to feel a little better.

The nurse’s reception was opposite the smoking room. Edward claimed most of the nurses did not care about them, he said they were only there for the money, because they could not get a job anywhere else. That there were only a few who really cared about you and wanted to help, the others saw them as an inconvenience to their working life, and did as little as they could to help any of the patients, and stayed in the office most of the time. Over time I began to understand Edward's thoughts, there were only certain nurses I bothered to speak to about Edward because they had some interest in the people there and wanted to help make their lives better, most sadly did not have this interest.

I never missed a day when I did not go and see him, some days he was pleased I was there- others he was quite hostile and dismissive. On days when he complied with the medication he would be very sleepy, and he would apologise and say he needed to sleep, and I would go. Nick often came with me and if he didn't Jane, Edwards's sister would join me. He was still very religious, and didn't trust the staff, sometimes furniture was pushed against his door, he was convinced he had been raped one night, and after that he refused medication because he wanted to be alert to what was happening. We often had really odd conversations it was difficult for me at times to go along with his train of thought, but Jane was more accepting than I. Nick also seemed to manage very strange conversations with him, that were very deep and a lot of sense was spoken by Edward, even though Edward was psychotic at the time.

I felt so helpless that I found it hard to take it all in, I loved him so much yet all my love could not help him. I took in fruit and tapes with his clean clothes on one visit. The following day his nurse told me he pushed all the clean clothes in a bin and squashed the fruit all over everything, she had kindly washed his clothes.

When I asked his consultant what he thought was wrong with Edward, he said he was not sure, and they were still assessing him. But he could not discuss Edward's condition or his medication due to confidentiality. I did ask if he thought his problem was drug induced. He said not, as the psychosis had lasted too long. He said this might be a one off bout of psychosis; he may come out of it and not have any more episodes. This conversation took place in the corridor by the stairs, not once was I asked to see the consultant in his office again because it was confidential, and I Edward's mother and main carer was not aloud to know. Yet I was the one that would be caring for him when he left hospital, but it seemed without any medical information on him.

When I asked Edward if there was anything he would like for Christmas, he said he wanted a white Reebok track suit, white Nike trainers with a gold tick, and a gold cross. I was amused that even in the very centre of this terrible illness he still wanted designer labels to wear.

The first week at the Warnford he was told about

the Mental Health Review Tribunal, where he may be able to get his sectioning lifted. He put in for one as soon as he heard about it, as he was convinced he was not ill, and was upset no one would accept he was the Son of God. I was really alarmed to hear about the Review and terrified they would lift the sectioning and he would leave the hospital. The staff did all they could to reassure me, they said no tribunal would lift the sectioning as he was desperately ill. He was hearing voices and responding to them, laughing and talking to himself. He wasn't complying with taking his medication regularly; neither was he responding to anyone. I had a letter to say the review would take place in the New Year as they were having trouble trying to find an independent doctor. I spoke to his solicitor twice; the first time she thought Edward was fine and wondered why he was in hospital. When she phoned me again she said she had just come from seeing Edward and she realised just how very ill he really was.

The oddest thing to all of this was they could only talk the case over with Adrian, as he was considered in law the responsible parent, due to the fact that he was a few years older than me. The fact that I had cared for Edward all his life and in everyway since the divorce including financially made no difference, I it seemed had no say on anything and neither could they discuss things with me. Even though they now called me his main carer.

On Christmas Eve he really upset his brother Jack, by telling him that his family meant nothing to him and we could all walk out and fall under a bus and be killed it would not bother him. Jack was devastated by this comment and really took it to heart, and I really felt for him, he was so upset as he thought the world of his little brother. I suggested Jack did not think of it as Edward speaking, but the illness. That if Edward had realised what he had said he would have been heart broken. I and Jane spent Christmas morning with him at the hospital, we gave him his presents, not a white track suit I couldn't find one, so I brought a light grey one, and the Nike trainers, he seemed very unimpressed with everything even the gold cross. I'm not even sure he realised it was Christmas Day. On my next visit his nurse told me he had given her all his gifts apart from the cross and asked her to give them to Oxfam. She had put them all in a bag and I took them home. Edward told me I should be proud that he had given his presents to charity. I had replied if I wished to give things to charity, I would choose the charity and what I gave. Things were rather cool between us for a few days after that.

On December the twenty seventh I received a letter saying the Tribunal would be held on Friday 29th at 10am. I was deeply shocked, as I had not expected anything to happen until after the New Year. I tried phoning Edwards solicitor but she was away for the Christmas break, another solicitor was going to sit in. I explained Edwards father was also away and I could not contact him, I explained he was the responsible parent. She said it didn't matter he didn't have to be there. When I spoke to the staff they were still sure everything would be all right, and that Edward was far too ill for any Tribunal to lift the sectioning. Edwards's consultant had told Adrian and I that he planned to put Edward onto section 3 if he did not start to comply with his medication in the next few days, I was desperate for my son to be well, and I wanted him to receive the medication to see if it would help.

The morning of the Tribunal Nick and I arrived over half an hour early, I felt sick and I couldn't stop shaking. There was concern because the independent doctor had not arrived, and he had not met Edward or even seen his notes. The doctor arrived just fifteen minuets before the start. At ten we were shown into a room on one side of a long table sat three people. Two men and one woman, they introduced them selves and that was the only time the women spoke. On the side where Nick and I were to sit was a young man I did not know, who explained Edwards CPN and social worker were both on leave so he was standing in for them. Next to him sat Nick, then myself, with Edward next to me, the stand in solicitor sat next to Edward and his consultant next to her. His consultant was concerned enough to break off his Christmas Leave to attend. The Chairman started the proceedings, but it was not long before the independent doctor took over the meeting completely.

Edwards's consultant gave a full report on Edwards's mental health, including observation of the nursing staff, even how he had been shouting and screaming the night before. He also read out a letter from Edwards GP who had also spent an hour with him the day before.

The night before this Review, Edward had decided to take his medication, and was very tired, and kept falling asleep, to the amusement of the independent doctor who kept laughing and saying "Your patients falling asleep doctor," to the consultant. When he was not doing that or speaking he sat with a slight smile on his face as if the whole proceedings were some kind of joke. I wanted to say, "This is my son's life you are dealing with, for Christ Sake take it seriously." But I kept quite I was in a place and a situation I knew nothing about. Near the end the doctor turned to me and said "I think you can take him home?" At that point I made the biggest and hardest decision I'd ever had to make before, and I refused to take him home, saying I did not feel he was well enough, that I felt he needed to be in hospital. After this we were asked to leave so the three people could make their decision.

The solicitor said it would take several hours and maybe we would like to get some fresh air. Edward sat on a chair outside the room and said "I'm staying here," so I sat with him. Nick said he'd go out for a cigarette and he went downstairs. The solicitor felt she had to stay with her client and stayed in the corridor, the consultant and the stand in CPN / social worker, stood away from us talking quietly. In less than ten minutes we were called back inside, we were not invited to sit down the independent doctor turned to the chairman with a smile. The Chairman said they felt that there was nothing wrong with Edward and he did not need to be held on section and he was free to go. For the first time in my fifty seven years I swore using the strongest swear words I knew very loudly in public, I told the three people exactly what I thought of them and left the room crying, I heard Edward say "What's wrong with mum." He was so unaware of what was happening around him. Nick heard me screaming and yelling from the bottom of the stairs. If that Mental Health Review Tribunal had been held at a later date with all Edward's mental health team there, and a decent independent doctor, the out come of what happened may have been completely different. If his sectioning had been upheld, he would have been moved up to section three, given medication, stayed in hospital until he was well enough to come home to Blewbury, where I would have cared for him, hopefully with a good mental health team supporting us. But some arrogant ill informed doctor who had no care about my son or his family decided to play God with my son's life.

It was just after this that Nick decided to pack up smoking, his timing I thought was really crap, but I was pleased he had decided to stop, though several months were hell, he constantly lost his temper often over nothing, and our house had a blue cloud of strong swear words hanging over it. There were several moments when I nearly ended things, I felt struggling to come to terms with my sons illness was bad enough, I just did not need more stress in my life, but we got through it some how.

Because I had refused to let Edward come home he had no where to go and he stayed in hospital until the beginning of March, during February he had heard from other patients that as a voluntary patient he could say he wanted to leave, and as he had no where to live, a place would be found for him. That's what he did he told his CPN he wanted to leave the hospital and he wanted to live in Oxford City.

NO TITLE

The thoughts manifest the word
The word manifests the deed,
The deed develops into habit
And habit hardens into character.
So watch the thought and its way with care,
And let it spring from love
Born out of concern for all beings.
As shadows follow the body
As we think so we become.

OXFORD

I had a phone call one bright March morning in 2001; it was from Edward's CPN to say Edward had left hospital. He had moved him into a bed and breakfast provided by the Council, just off the Cowley Road in Oxford. He explained Edward had no money and he had lent him ten pounds. I was really alarmed I knew Edward was still not very well and also very vulnerable. Adrian and I went out there straight away to see him. We found him upstairs in a seedy house that once had been a family home; all the rooms had been made into bed and breakfast rooms. Edward was sitting on a bed in a dingy little room; I suspect he had been in that position since he had arrived he looked sad, lost, and very lonely. I think he was completely bewildered by where he was and what was happening to him.

The single bed was against the far wall from the door, a window was in that wall that looked out on an over grown back garden full of junk. At the foot of the bed on the other wall was a washbasin that you had to kneel on the bed to use. A grubby mirror was above that, next to that was a wall cupboard dating from the fifties painted white, the sliding door did not work due to over painting, and so it remained open. Then a chimneybreast jutted out with a blocked off fireplace. The wall by the door had an old double wardrobe against it, the hanging rail was broken, but the shelving gave space to put things, again the door to this was hanging off. The wall with the door had a kitchen chair against it and a new fridge, the only thing that looked clean. The bedding was faded and looked grubby. There were no eating utensils; I went down stairs to inspect the kitchen. There was a cooker, no other furniture in the room apart from a small table, no cupboards, work surfaces, or cooking utensils, not even a kitchen sink. Next to that room was the bathroom. The bath had lost most of its enamel and I knew Edward would never use it. The toilet was filthy and smelt the hand basin not much cleaner.

The first thing I did was go down the Cowley Road with Edward and brought him everything he needed to set up a home, when it became clear he was determined to stay there. We also stocked up on food, this went into the fridge, and Nick gave him a microwave when we discovered he did not want to use the cooker downstairs. After that I scrubbed out the toilet and basin, I kept a check on these once a week. His sister and I brought posters for his wall and a rug we saw in Oxfam that we knew he would like.

I had still not returned to work, I was suffering from a stress related illness due to coping with Edward's illness and had been signed off by my doctor, it was a very much needed time because I needed to go to Oxford every day to check on Edward, who was still very ill, and unable to care for himself. As I do not drive this was a very difficult task at times.

Though he had applied for income support and invalidity benefit, this had been all organised by the hospital before he left, he received nothing for sixteen weeks, and if it had not been for me keeping him supplied with food and money while he insisted on staying at the B&B, he would have starved to death. How others manage in the same situation, without a family or friends to support them I dread to think. On his second day at Oxford I called in on him in the afternoon with Jane, his CPN was there and was telling Edward about a drop- in centre at Temple Cowley, and he also told him he needed to get his medical certificate down to the benefits office so his benefits could be arranged, he was also given an address of a local GP where he had to go and register.

Edward took all this information and appeared positive towards his CPN, and gave the impression he would be able to do it. Once he had left Edward turned to me and asked if I understood where the

Drop in Centre was, he was nervous about going and looking for it, and asked us to help him. Jane said "Come on I know where he means, I'll take you in the car, but it is near enough to walk so don't worry."
That day we took him to Temple Cowley, showed him his local shops and the Drop in Centre. He did try the Drop in Centre several times, but most of the people there were elderly and were people with learning disabilities and Edward felt out of place and uncomfortable so he did not continue to attend.

The next day Nick and I took him to the benefits office so he could drop in his medical certificate, and then he asked if we could take him to OXPEN's the local college of farther education. He wanted an application form, he still wanted to take his A- levels and apply to an Art College. He'd filled it in so when I saw him next we went through the form together before we posted it. Over the next few weeks Nick and I kept phoning the benefits office to find out why Edward was not receiving any help. By now I was on no pay with the company I worked for having been off work for so long, and things were becoming difficult. At one point Edward had a letter asking him to call into the benefits office, again Nick and I took him. This time they said they needed a medical certificate; Edward tried to tell them he had given them one, and even described the person he had given it too. But they claimed they had not received it, and Edward felt intimidated by their attitude towards him and walked out.

Next was to get him registered with the local doctor his CPN had told him about, once that was done I took his new medical certificate into the benefits office. Weeks went past and no response to none of the letters I sent, or the endless phone calls we kept making. Nick at one point was on the phone to them for one whole afternoon trying to sort it out. In the mean time we kept Edward supplied with food, he brought his washing home every weekend and showered whenever he visited me. I saw him most days at times when I could not visit him I spoke to him on the phone. He use to come home most weekends, still no benefits had been sorted out, and though I still felt unwell I knew I had to return to work. In one last hope I wrote to Edward's MP Boris Johnson explaining how long Edward had been out of hospital, how ill he was and that it was becoming very difficult to financially support him. I received a letter from Boris Johnson promising to look into it and within a week Edward's benefits were available. The large back payment Edward received was too much for Edward to handle in his present state. In the room next to him was an older man who had drink related problems, he had befriended Edward soon after he had moved in, and kept an eye on him. With all that money they went out on drinking binges, and Edward met his son who started him smoking cannabis again.
In the mean time I had received letters from agents of Edward's last flat in London, demanding rent. This took several months to sort out, and endless nasty letters were sent to me, that became very threatening near the end. It was impossible to

speak to anyone by phone, things began to get very nasty, and the threats started to become very personal and I became quite frightened by their attitude. In the end I had to seek help from a solicitor. Adrian around this time started dealing with the £900.00 fine and the courts. Eventually the fine and court records were dropped due to Edward's mental state. Some how my solicitor managed to stop the awful threatening letters to me, and the whole thing died down.

The signs of Edward smoking cannabis did not start straight away, he had been given an interview date with OXPENS College. He had to take a portfolio of his artwork, and has he had destroyed his most recent work. I searched through drawings he had given me over time, and he did a few more sketches' to add to it. His talent was still there though it exhausted him doing them. He managed to go to the interview and to his joy he was accepted, I felt so pleased for him and proud that he had managed the interview.

Over this time I was becoming increasingly worried about my son, I hated him living in that awful room, the landlord received £200.00 a week from the council for that little room alone, yet none of the money this person received ever went into making the house more pleasant for those living there. Every Monday the occupants of the house had to walk down to the landlord several streets away, where they were given a packet of cereal, a pint of milk, and a loaf of bread and some spread, this was breakfast for seven days. Several times over this period I phoned the Samaritans, desperate to talk to someone. Around this time I phoned a mental health help line too as I was feeling really down and desperate about my son. I needed to find out more about mental illness, they put me in touch with the National Schizophrenia Fellowship (now called Rethink) and a Coordinator working in Oxford.

The first time I saw her I cried for most of my visit, she understood my fears for Edward and empathised with how I felt. She gave me so much information, and literature I could understand, she told me about various projects that could help Edward, including a football group that was run for young mentally ill people. She advised me to speak to his CPN, as Edward would have to be referred by him to the various projects. (though I asked his CPN to help Edward enter various places he had shown interest in, and he said he would, he never did manage to organise anything, this man was so over worked he eventually became very ill himself.)

She also said she would look into finding some sort of support housing for him; she was very aware how vulnerable Edward was living in a bed and breakfast. She gave me lots of information on all aspects of mental illness, and for the first time I felt there was some positive hope for us. I returned to work with a more positive out look, and the Co-ordinator kept in touch with me, and both Nick and I saw her on several occasions and each time I felt more positive about the future. She also mentioned that both Nick and I should have been given a carer's assessment and that she would contact the Oxfordshire Mental Health Team dealing with Edward and arrange one for us.

We had had a visit from a young social worker when Edward first went into hospital, in December 2000. She was friendly and kind, she gave us a web site so we could down load information on schizophrenia, it was a very thick medical document a lot of it was repeated, and so long it was difficult to read. The parts I read I understood but because it was written for medical people I found it hard to retain, and really required something written in laymen's terms. The web site was given after I requested information on metal illness; she seemed unable to explain it herself. It was this young woman that returned to do the assessment, she seemed little more that a child herself, and I found it odd to be assessed by her. But she was a sweet person and I went along with the questioning, as did Nick.

When her report came back I was shocked to see how little she had listened or maybe understood. She had us down as husband and wife and Nick as Edward's stepfather, and that he was financially responsible for Edward. There were many other minor mistakes, which I ignored, but I did phone her about the mistake of us being married and Nick being financially responsible as he never was, all the way through the time he knew Edward. He was my son and I took that financial responsibility.

When I explained she just laughed, I was already stressed with Edward's illness and her immaturity of dealing with my complaint did not help my feelings, but upset me further. I wrote and complained, now maybe I would have acted different, but at that time I was not myself and very concerned about my son, and she was the social worker in the Mental Health Caring Team, I expected a little more than laughter, maybe I expected too much. Things were never the same after that and she never kept in contact or spoke to us again.

In the mean time Edward sadly continued to drink heavily and smoke cannabis, one weekend at the end of June I asked him if he would mind staying over on the Saturday to look after the dogs, while I and Nick were away for the night. We had been invited to a wedding and were going to stay over night; at the time of asking Edward seemed all right. I left him a prepared meal, and plenty of things for breakfast; I locked any alcohol in the garden shed, for Edward's own safety. I did phone him on Saturday afternoon and he sounded fine.

On our return Sunday morning I knew as soon as I saw him something was wrong. He was sitting on the sofa looking very down. First thing he said was "I've had a bit of an accident mum, sorry."
I enquired what was wrong; he told me he had knocked an expensive limited edition bowl off the table, and that it had broke. Though I was upset, at first I accepted what had happened as an accident,

and told him not to worry. But then I saw a china paperweight was also missing, and that was from the mantelshelf and I was puzzled. I went out to the dustbin to see if the pieces of the bowl could be repaired, and I discovered it had been smashed into tiny bits, along with the paperweight. I also discovered it had been broken out on the patio; in fact I'm still finding odd bits of it to this very day. I realised it was far from an accident, I also discovered in the bin his dinner I had left him untouched, a video tape of Eminem that had been broken and several other rapper tapes also destroyed. He also told me he had gone for a walk and had lost the front door key.

I don't think I handled the whole thing very well, I told him I knew he had smashed the things on purpose, that I was very hurt and upset. I asked him why he was so angry with me, and what I had done to deserve such a reaction from him. I told him I felt he should go back to his room. He was very remorseful and upset by what he had done, and he said sorry several times. When we dropped him off at his room in Cowley he said again he was sorry and that he loved me, and he did look very upset and in need of a hug, but I ignored my instinct to hug him and walked away. I told him I still loved him but I needed a little space away from him for a while, and that I would talk to him in the morning. Nick managed to keep out of it though I knew he was very angry by what had happened. We talked over the episode for days wandering what had gone on in our absence. The dogs were very subdued for a while and our neighbour said he had played music until the early hours and that she had heard him moving about and banging doors all night. We had to have the lock changed on the front door, as we had no real idea what had happened to the front door key. Edward spoke of it several months later and I explained to him that the bowl had a sentimental meaning to Nick and I, but it was over with now and not to worry it was after all only a china bowl. We did hug then.

This episode was recorded in Edward's notes as an assault on his mother, when I read this after his death on the investigation report I asked the mental health people to change it, as it was not true, he had never assaulted me, he'd smashed some objects and that was all. What they then added to the notes was "Edward's mother and father now state this assault did not take place, and have asked for this information to be taken out of this report." The comments on him assaulting me still remain in the report.

Not long after this Edward's brother Jack opened up his own business in Cheltenham. He was opening an antique rug and carpet shop. He had been in the business since leaving school, and was very knowledgeable; he'd been talking about starting his own shop for sometime. I encouraged him believing it was a good thing to try while he was young, and that if he did not try it he would regret it in later years. He was very excited about the project and one morning myself Jane and

Edward were to travel with Jack to see the shop and I was going to treat them to lunch after.

The night before Edward rang to say he did not want to come, then suddenly at nine the next morning he said he did want to come, I said we'd pick him up on the way. Fifteen minuets after that call he rang again to find out where we were I told him we had not left yet and gave him a time to expect us. When we arrived at his house I knew he was very ill again, he looked all around before he fully came out of the door. Then he pulled up his hood over his baseball hat and ran to the car, looking really scared. He sat in the front with Jack and Jane and I sat in the rear, the whole of the journey Edward talked to himself and laughed, not loud enough for anyone to hear what he was saying, but loud enough to know he was troubled. When we arrived at Cheltenham Edward refused to leave the car, so we three had a quick looked around, but we were all worried about leaving Edward too long, and I felt sorry for Jack as it was not such a good day for him as it should have been.

We parked the car in a multi-story car park and again Edward refused to leave the car, so I rushed off to buy some sandwiches and drinks for everyone. When Edward did talk he explained he stayed over at his fathers and that his father had injected him in the leg with something. We all told him we did not think his father would do that and why would he, but Edward was adamant it had happened. As we drove back Edward started to laugh again, and Jack asked him to share the joke, and Edward became quite hostile towards him. So Jack apologised and we all travelled home in silence apart from the mumblings from Edward.

The following morning I phoned Edward's CPN and told him about the day before and how worried I was about Edward. He phoned me back sometime later and said he'd been round to see Edward, but he would not come to the door and he was not answering his phone. He told me not to worry that he had arranged for a doctor to come and see him. I also spoke to someone from the NSF I explained how Edward had been on the trip to Cheltenham that he was talking to himself and laughing. They said that as he did not seem to be a threat to himself or anyone else, he was fine and probably very happy hearing voices and talking to them. My argument was if he had been born hearing voices and responding to them, then yes it would be fine, as that would be part of him. But this was a sign that he was becoming ill, again it was quoted that he was not a danger to himself or anyone else, and I said, "Surely by then it could be too late?"

NO TITLE

All is still and calm,
Nobody doing any harm,
When all of a sudden
Hats and newspapers fly
Way up in the sky.
Trees whistle in the wind
And everybody rushes in.
Suddenly everything falls down
As the wind slowly dies.
Then there was a quiet sound
Not at all loud
I realise its coming from a cloud
'Pardon me it say's'
How disgusting.

SECTION THREE

In the end it was his consultant from the hospital that called to see Edward with his CPN. He was assessed, again the police had to be called and he was hand cuffed and taken back into hospital under section three of the Mental Health Act. He was very ill and suffering delusions. On this second admission we were told Edward was suffering with Paranoia Schizophrenia. Of course his benefits stopped the day he entered hospital, funny how quick they can act at times.

Edward was angry with me; he blamed me for him being admitted into hospital again, and said he did not want to see me. I felt very upset at this and found it very hard, but I respected his request and only kept in touch via the hospital staff. Then one day a few weeks later he phoned me and asked why hadn't I been to see him. So again I was back visiting every day, it made it very tiring as I was at work all day and then travelled onto the hospital before going home. I heard he had already put in for a Mental Health Review and the old fear from the last one crept into me again and I started to worry. I talked to the NSF Co-coordinator in Oxford again about my fears; I also talked about my feelings of not letting him come home after the last Tribunal Review, I felt guilty and as if I had rejected my son, by refusing to let him come home. She said that for many people with schizophrenia it was less stressful for them to live by themselves. That it was often stress that led to a relapse of their illness, that they were very sensitive to a change in atmosphere. Edward had always been a sensitive person even when a small boy and I had been aware he was even more sensitive now. I learnt so much from this person, and she was so understanding I will always be indebted to her.

At first Edward did not want me to attend his next Mental Health Review Tribunal, I felt upset, but again accepted his request. The medical staff of his ward approached me and asked me to write to the Tribunal and ask them for this Review to be held correctly. I did this and reminded them of what happened at the first one, even though I had no idea what a Mental Health Review Tribunal was or how it was run, I did know the independent doctor should have spent far more time reading Edward's notes and should have interviewed my son, before the review.

The day before the Review was to take place Edward asked me to be there, as I was about to leave we hugged and I could feel the fear in him. It was often like this when I hugged him now, he was so scared I could feel him shake and he would cling to me. I hated leaving him feeling like that and I felt so helpless, I wanted to take away his pain, for him to have his youth back. Sometimes I would see young people his age having fun and enjoying life, and my heart would break because my son should have been doing the same. I wanted so much to help him get his life back but I could not help him I could only love him and this I did with all my heart and soul.

On the day of the review I was shown into a large room down stairs in the hospital. Everyone who should have been there was there, plus his named nurse and deputy, the independent doctor had been to see Edward twice and spent several hours with him. The chair-person remained in charge of the whole proceedings, and everyone at the Review was asked for their own feelings on Edward's mental health, including Edward. The whole proceedings were held like an official hearing, everyone was heard and their thoughts respected. What ever the out come I could not have found fault with the way it was held. We did not know the result of the Hearing until the following

day, when it had been decided to keep Edward on Section Three of the Mental Health Act, as he was not complying with his medication.
After that he was given Depo injections, he had been prescribed Risperdone when he was first admitted, but this did not agree with him so it changed to Olanzapene which he hated as it made him fat, at nineteen he was very concerned about his appearance, he'd also read on the notes in the box the medication came in, about the side effects - one of them being a loss of libido. Something else a young man of nineteen did not want to happen. He also hated feeling like a zombie, he felt his own thoughts and feelings were buried deep inside him and he was unable to express himself because the medication took him over. This was some of the reasons why he hated to take his medication, though the main one was the simple fact he did not want to be ill and could not accept it, and he hated the word schizophrenia. I use to say it's just a word it explains an illness, it can be called anything you want, because it's not what you are, you are still Edward. But it was hard for me to get my head round it at times, so I knew it was ten times harder for Edward.

Edward only liked family to visit him and declined seeing anyone else even two of his close friends Harry and Tim, who asked to visit him but he refused to see them. I also contacted Katy and she rang him several times but again he would not see her. Something I did discover because I was very open about Edward and his illness, as I was never ashamed of him suffering from schizophrenia, in fact I was quite proud of the way he battled with it. I told people who asked after him what was wrong, it was then I discovered how many people I knew and had known for sometime had a member of the family who suffered from mental illness, and in one case suffered themselves, and I had know this person for twenty years and never knew until Edward went into hospital.

From time to time while Edward was in hospital they held what they called Care Meetings. Myself, Nick and Edward's father were always asked to be present, Edward would be there with his named nurse, his CPN and his social worker and his psychiatrist chaired it. Some meetings were stressful, others quite productive, they mostly depended on Edward's moods, how unwell he was and what he happened to be feeling at that particular time. At one meeting he walked out and sat on the floor outside the door, but the psychiatrist continued with the meeting, which I found rather odd as it was to find out what was best and helpful for Edward, and he was not there to hear or have any input.

Something that was brought up at every meeting was the fact that we lived in Blewbury, this village was on the boarders of Oxfordshire and Berkshire, the Thames Mental Health Team who catered for Oxfordshire who were caring for Edward at this time, thought Edward should be looked after by the Wallingford Mental Health Team, who came under

Berkshire. There were always long discussions on this; I would remind them that Edward was living in Oxford and not Reading. This it seemed was also a problem as Thames Team did not really cover Oxford City, I'd ask why he couldn't come under Oxford City and it seemed the Thames Team managed the Warnford Hospital. I grew very tired of this, and almost felt guilty for living in the wrong place. I have discovered since that someone living on the boarders of two counties are called "Overlaps" and that it seems is what my son was and why it was so difficult to get the correct medical help he needed, because he was an "Overlap" he'd have received better help if he had been an alien. What I will never understand what the fuck did it matter. They had a young man seriously mentally ill, where he lived was immaterial he required help, for goodness sake, but like everything it comes down to money before people.

One of the other things I found really strange sitting in on these meetings was how the psychiatrist decided what were facts and what were delusions when Edward said something. Some were obvious such as being the Son of God, or being the devil, or a famous rapper, but other things he said were not so obvious, I'd known him for twenty years and was never completely sure on some comments. My son was an intelligent young man, and even when very psychotic he knew how to string someone along, and tell them what he thought they wanted to hear. I use to watch him play games with the psychiatrist, and for the great doctor to be drawn in. Ed would laugh about the meetings after and tell Nick and me how stupid the doctors were, and how they believed what he said, "I just tell them what they want to hear." he use to say to us.

Some times Edward was asked about what he wanted for the future, he would speak of his ambition to attend college and study art, and one day make animated films, this they considered was a delusion, and they would question this. But when he said he'd find a job in McDonalds, they saw this as real. A theme he spoke of every time we had a meeting due to the fact that he felt the staff wanted to hear him speak of something with a lower expectation. He would tell me this later after the meeting. This comment was written down as fact and what he wanted to aspire too. Even my saying he was a talented artist did not change their view of him attending art school as a delusion, it seems they only felt him fit to work in McDonalds, nothing wrong with that, but I knew he was capable of more as Edward did.

The other thing he insisted that happened was the rape when he was at sixth form college, and in the hospital. This they had no doubt was a delusion, never any question about that, but when he said he had injected heroin, that was fact, even though Edward had a fear of injections, one of the reasons the consultant had admitted him to hospital a second time was because he was convinced his father had been injecting him in the leg when he stayed with him. Always when he started to become psychotic Edward would talk about his fear of injections and accuse someone of sticking needles into him. When Edward said about injecting heroin I felt he said it to shock, he was in that sort of mood. They believed he took crack and L.S.D. it's possible he had tried it at some time, I don't know but he was not a regular user, I saw him most days and when he stayed with us in Blewbury he was certainly clean. They believed he drank twenty pints of larger at a time, this I do know was not possible, after four or five pints in our local with us, he had trouble walking back home, tripping over nothing and walking into walls. No one will ever really know what was true and what were delusions now, but I still wondered how they could judge at the time.

The depo injection seemed to be having a good effect, Edward was permitted to go out for a few hours at first, and we'd go into Oxford, usually HMV or Virgin store where he'd spend his time looking through rap and heavy metal and Rock CDs. Eventually they would let him home to Blewbury for a day, and then for the weekend. Though he was often very exhausted by these outings he seemed to be coming out of the psychosis, it was like seeing a butterfly emerge from a chrysalis, and his sense of humour was coming back, a great sign for me, especially when he could laugh at himself. At home he helped me paint a garden wall and Nick put up a green house and life seemed to be taking on a positive air again. He went on an outing with the hospital to a wildlife park, one week-day, there he brought me a picture of a tiger with her cubs, and it had written on the bottom, "A loving family is hard to beat." Even now looking at it or just remembering brings me to tears.

The hospital had a laundry at first Edward used this, but his clothes started to disappear. He and I searched the lost property box, and the laundry room but none of his clothes were there. I asked several of the nursing staff, but they showed no interest or offered any help. After that we decided I would collect his washing once a week and do it at home. It was not only his clothes that disappeared, but books and CDs as well. None of these were ever found and it was not the lack of searching on Edward's part, he found this very upsetting and hated the lack of interest from the nursing staff. He felt because he was mentally ill it did not matter if his personal things were taken that his illness made him nothing, and this made him angry, me too I must confess.

South Park in Oxford is very close to the Warnford Hospital and every August they have what they call Music in The Park. A large stadium is built and a free concert is put on for anyone who wants to go. Edward had asked his named nurse if he could go, some of the other people in the ward were able to attend, and he wanted to join them. His named nurse said he could, but on the Sunday of the concert his named nurse was not on duty, and he was not aloud to go with the others. He phoned me very upset as Samantha Mumba was appearing and he really had a big thing about her. I phoned the hospital and asked if I go with him and they agreed, his sister said she would come to. We collected Edward the concert had only just started and we had only missed a couple of acts. This was Edward's first time in a large crowd and at times he became very pale and we would encourage him to sit down until he felt better. At first he was worried that he had missed Samantha Mumba, but the presenters eventually listed all those who were to appear still and her name was mentioned much to Ed's joy. She did not appear until seven thirty, but it was well worth the wait to see the pleasure on his face and many others in the crowd.

One night at about ten a.m. not long after the concert Edward phoned me, he was in tears, "I am mentally ill aren't I mum?" I told him it was true he was mentally ill, we talked for awhile but I was unable to comfort him over the phone, and I had to fight back my tears as we spoke and keep calm, so I could be of help to him. As soon as he rang off I phoned the nurses station, and asked one of the nurses to go to him I explained how upset he was and I felt he needed to talk. One of the younger nurses, whom I found had a certain amount of empathy for the people in their care, went to him and spent time with him, until he was feeling calmer and able to go to bed.

WHY NOT

If I could blame who I wanted to blame,
And if they could accept with a smile,
Maybe not their fault,
Maybe not even to do with them.
Then they could blame me
Just for the sake of it.

OUT OF HOSPITAL

Well Again.
As September drew closer Edward's time to start College was getting nearer, I asked his CPN if any one in his Mental Health Team had contacted the college to tell them about Edward. When he said no I contacted them myself and explained he was at the moment in hospital but getting better every day. I could see the improvement in him; he was like his old self and feeling very positive. I met the college nurse and we had a talk and then we made an appointment for Ed' to meet him. He showed him a room next to his office where he could go any time he felt pressured or stressed. He felt Edward trying to do three A -levels was too much and tried to persuade him to do Key Skills. Edward was adamant he wanted to do A Levels.

A week before he started college a Care Meeting was arranged, they wanted him to remain in hospital but said they had found him a place in support housing in Cholsey, a village about five miles away from Blewbury, still in Oxfordshire. Edward was very pleased about the support housing, but not remaining in hospital until he moved to Cholsey. He did not want to be in a mental hospital while attending college. I asked if he could come home until the sheltered accommodation was ready and it was agreed he could do that. He was to remain on section three until the next meeting in October. Because they were moving him to Cholsey, they were also going to transfer him to the Fair Mile Mental Health Hospital in Cholsey and he would have a new consultant and Mental Health Team. The Thames Team were to get their way at last and transfer him over to a Berkshire Mental Health Team. Edward seemed happy with this, and they were to arrange the transfer as soon as they could. His benefits needless to say took months to come through and another letter to Boris Johnson before any signs of it appeared again.

A couple of days before he started college we went into Reading to buy him some clothes. We had a really great day, he was happy and wanted to choose things and try them on. We had an enjoyable lunch and talked and laughed a lot, it was one of the best times I had spent with him for a few years. I think we were both feeling very positive about the future. It had been so long since I had seen my son so relaxed and happy; he was laughing and joking that day. I saw a skirt in a shop window and he even persuaded me to go in and try it on, and he waited quite content and not at all stressed or agitated. It was really a lovely day and I felt very hopeful for the future.

On his first day at college he returned home worrying because he was in a class for A level art with all girls there was not any other male in the class, even the teacher was a female. He found it so difficult he walked out of the second lesson and dropped the subject. The two other subjects he had decided to take had huge great gaps between the lessons one first thing in the morning the other last one in the afternoon, both on Mondays and Tuesdays. His worry was what to do between those lessons, we tried to find out if there was a common room or library, but both of us found it difficult to find any one to help. I phoned the college nurse in the end but he was hard to speak too and I kept leaving messages. He made an appointment with Edward. But they never met up, first the nurse was off sick, then when another appointment was made, Ed' said the nurse never showed up.

On his second day at college he came home and used Nick's razor to shave his head, he'd also spent his lunch money having his ears pierced again. This is how he had looked at sixteen before he started six-form college. On his return from college after he had done this he was very upset and wished he hadn't done it. I think he was trying to go back, trying to start again from before his life started to go wrong for him. I felt so sad and didn't know how to help him feel better. At that time as I was cooking our supper he suddenly said "Mum do you think I will ever be able to live a normal life?"

I replied "Yes I do believe it is possible, things are better than they were several months ago. I'm really proud of the way you are handling things. I think if you keep taking your medication, lay off of cannabis things will improve, it's just going to take time Ed', we have to be patient."

He smiled and I returned to the cooking, I did not realize then that he had already stopped taking his medication. He'd had his last depo injection the day he left hospital, and had been given 1.5 mg of Haloperidol to take twice a day one in the evening and one in the mornings.

Over September and the first three weeks of October things went really well, he moved into the sheltered housing in Cholsey. The Warden Dan was a really nice guy who was a trained psychiatric nurse, he had part time help of a care assistant Holly. There were eight people in the house two older men. Who I was told were long term residents and five other young men around Edward's age, all with similar problems. Ed' was happy to be with people of his own age group and soon made friends with a lad called Chris. Selsea Place was two houses knocked together, with a main shared sitting room with main TV shared kitchen/dinning room, that all so housed a pool table. Each had their own rooms with TV, fridge, sink, bed, armchair, dressing table, chest of drawers and cupboard. There were a couple of bathrooms on each floor. It was nicely decorated, and the kitchen area was modern and clean, though the sitting room always looked untidy, it was nicely furnished.

On Monday and Tuesdays he attended college, every Wednesday after work I met up with him and we went out for a meal, some times joined by Nick, Jane or Jack. Thursday Nick use to pick him up in the afternoon and Ed' would help Nick in the grounds where he was an Estate Manager for fifty six homes for the elderly. He'd stay over night and help Nick again on Friday, and Nick would pay him at the end of the day. On Saturday he would either stay with me until Sunday, or choose to spend the weekend with his father. Jane would always visit if he was at home. Things were beginning to settle into a routine and Edward seemed to cope with it and appeared happy.

Because the house in Blewbury was only two bedrooms Nick and I decided to borrow some money to have an extension built onto the side of the house, where we would have a new kitchen and above it another bedroom. This would mean Edward could have his own room and we would still have a spare bedroom for grandchildren or guests who wished to stay. I felt that though Edward may not want to live with us full time, but there would always be a place he could come to when needed. A place where he could store anything and it would be untouched. When the plans were drawn up I showed them to him, and he seemed pleased that he would have a base when he needed it. He often used to ask if he was a burden to me. I never felt he was, he was my son and I was there for all my children, whatever their need or problem. I always told him he never was a burden, and I hoped him having a permanent position in Blewbury for whenever he needed it and not having to sleep downstairs if someone came to stay would help him feel more secure.

At the end of October Nick and I were due to go on holiday and I would miss his next Care Meeting. His Thames CPN was still seeing him as they had not heard from the Wallingford Mental Health Team yet, or the Fair Mile Mental Hospital even though contact had been made several times by the Thame team. Adrian said he would be at the Care Meeting and Jane said she would keep in touch with Edward while I was a way, I hoped his father would as well. When I told Edward what I was doing he said "Good you deserve a holiday mum." While I was away Jane did keep in touch and also took him out for a meal and to the cinema.

Nick and I did not have a good holiday in Malta, it was messed up by Nick secretly starting to smoke, this made him feel bad and so he was short tempered again. It did not help that money was also short and at one point the bank stopped us drawing money out of cash points. It took several phone calls by me to the UK to sort things out.

On my return from Malta I discovered Edward's CPN had gone on long term sick leave, that his section three had been lifted, though he remained an enhanced patient "what ever that meant." That Edward had started to smoke cannabis again, and all the negative symptoms of his illness were returning. Without his CPN to talk things over with and no Mental Health Team, I contacted Thame to find out when the Fair Mile were going to take over, and discovered they were still waiting for a reply. Edward had given up going to college, did not want to continue to help Nick and did not want to meet up and go out with me on a Wednesdays.

On November the eighth it was Edward's Birthday I took him to Reading after work to buy some new trainers. This trip was completely different to our last one, as I'm only five foot one and he was six foot I had to run to keep up with him. We flashed through shoe and sports shops so quickly, people stopped to look at us. We must have presented a comical sight, Ed' in a bandana and base ball cap on top, in very baggy clothes not only due to fashion but weight loss too, with an elderly short chubby clapped out mum in tow, trying to keep up. He knew exactly what he wanted and would scan the rows of shoes on the shelves, then turn and walk out with out a word. At times I had just about caught up with him as he turned to leave. When we had at last found what he wanted he refused to try them on and waited outside while I paid for them. After that he insisted on going back to Cholsey, where he said "thanks" and shot out the car and back to the safety of his room.

In December Edward had a bad night, possibly due to drink or cannabis or both he got into a fight with one of the other residents who had also been drinking, and a coffee table was broken. Edward owned up to it and was given a warning that any more trouble and he would be evicted, he also had to pay for the broken table. I did not help him on this he had to work it out for himself and paid so much each time he received his benefits.

Christmas of 2001 Edward came to us on Christmas Eve to stay over possibly until New Year, if his father was not going to see him. The Cholsey house was unattended until New Year and apart from the two older guys most of the people were going to relatives or friends. Edward's friend Chris had been admitted into the Fair Mile earlier in the month the cannabis both had been smoking was having it's affect. As he and Ed' were not sleeping any more and were keeping other people awake, they were both becoming unwell. But Chris had a mental health team, his needs were being taken care of. Edward on the other hand was in limbo land he was neither a Warnford's patient any more or the Fair Miles. I often spoke to Dan over this time as he was as worried as I about what was not happening, to help Edward. He also felt very strongly that Edwards's medication was not strong enough, and not the right sort, that it was just keeping him above psychosis.

During November Nick and I had attended a Carer's Course run by the Oxford C0-Ordinator of the N.S.F. This proved to be very beneficial not only by meeting others with mentally sick relatives, but by hearing what should be out there to help careers and users. A pharmacist spoke of all the medications available and possible side effects. Here I learnt Edward was on one of the old type of drugs and that there were more modern and often better kinds. We learnt the best way to help a person when they were delusional. At one point we were told to face someone and hold a conversation, this I did, and some one came up behind me and whispered horrible insulting things in my ear, not only did I find the words disturbing it was very difficult to concentrate on the conversation I was trying to have. This it was explained was what it was like for some people all day long. For me it had only lasted a few moments and I was troubled, how I would cope with weeks of it I don't know, I'm not sure I could. I learnt so much from these classes I realized the health care my son was receiving, was even worse than I suspected.

Christmas, Edward was really ill; he kept earphones all day and night because of the voices. This was when he told me he hadn't taken his medication since September; again I don't know how true this was. I went with Edward to the Midnight Service at Blewbury Church, even though I could see the voices were bothering him, he enjoyed being in church and taking communion with me. I was really happy I shared that moment with him. Nick and I had hardly any sleep on Christmas Eve due to Edward moving about constantly at night. Jane who was also with us had the same trouble, so Christmas day we were all exhausted, and Edward spent the day with the ear phones on. I phoned his father on Boxing Day asking if he was going to spend any time with Edward over the holiday period. He said no, but he did manage to speak to him on the phone. As he was not seeing any other members of the family during the week between Christmas and the New Year, Nick and I had him over every day but took him back at night so we could sleep. We were always invited to Jacks on Christmas Eve for a drink and to exchange presents, this was where the very last photo was ever taken of Edward, Christmas Eve 2001 at Jacks and Louise's house.

Just after New Year Edward's father called to say Ed' had called him for a lift to Maidenhead as his girl friend was very ill in a hospital I explained he did not have a girl friend, and to leave it until the morning. I said to explain to Edward if she was that ill she would only be allowed to see close relatives. The following morning when I spoke to Edward it seemed the problem was solved and she was out of intensive care, and was leaving hospital that day. He never spoke of this again.

Over the next two months Edward became more and more detached he hardly saw or spoke to anyone. In desperation I contacted the Thames Team asking for help, they arranged a meeting in Thames. At this meeting it was suggested Edward went back onto Depo Injections and he agreed.

Sadly they did not have the medication there so they could not do it straight away. Dan arranged for an appointment with his GP and again when they saw the doctor he did not have the medication on hand so once more it was not done. By the time the medication was available it was too late Edward was too far gone and refused to have it.

In desperation I wrote to the Wallingford Mental Health Team at the beginning of February asking what I had to do to get help for my son, this letter was used against me by the Wallingford Mental Health Team at the inquest. The letter resulted in a Care Meeting being arranged for the 28th of February at 10-00 to be held at the Fair Mile Hospital. Here I met his new consultant for the first time, though he was surprised to find Edwards family there, he was a younger doctor than his previous one, who was new to the Mental Health Care in England as he had been working in Scotland. He had already met Edward and he felt Edward was too ill to attend the meeting and asked him to remain outside in the waiting room.

Big mistake! At this meeting was his new CPN “a stuck up cow” who wanted nothing to do with Edward’s relatives being involved with his care, and did her utmost to ignore us. As his consultant started to say he was very concerned about Edwards’s condition and that he wanted to bring him into hospital straight away to stabilize him and sort out his medication. The new CPN and a social worker from Thames, who had offered me support and an ear during his time in limbo, both said

"You can't do that."

The Doctor looked puzzled and said "he clearly needs help," they then quoted the danger to himself or others as a reason why he could not be taken into hospital. At this point Edward came into the room; he announced he had no intentions of going into hospital, and that he was perfectly fit, there was nothing wrong with him but that we all needed medical help. His consultant calmed him down and asked him if he would just come into hospital for two weeks, so he could help sort out his medication. Edward refused the consultant then asked everyone apart from Edward to wait outside. While sitting in the waiting room I tried to talk to his new CPN She clearly did not want to talk to me and basically snubbed me, and though I was sitting next to her, she turned so her back was towards me, and I felt dismissed.

After a few moments Edward walked out of the consultant's office and left the hospital. We were called back into the office and he said "I guess we have to wait until he crashes then?"
To which the other two mental health staff agreed, it was then decided that the next meeting with Edward would be at the end of May, and his new CPN would call in and see him when he required a visit. I left feeling very let down and that my son was still in limbo. As far as I could see Edward was not going to request a visit from his new CPN as he

did not know her, and she seemed far colder person to his last CPN who was a very caring guy, who had been with Edward since the beginning of December 2000, when he was first admitted to hospital. They had grown to know each other, and he knew how to handle Edward at his most awkward times.

NO TITLE

A sudden peace, sudden relief
Deep down inside finally free,
So simple, could it really be this easy?
Take one step forward, now no turning back.
This time forever with no turning track.
Once again I've stumbled to my feet
The generalization makes things so neat.
A sighing of hope
It's been too long sliding on soap.
Looking back I finally see,
It's all experience maybe bad, but behind me.
I can comfortably sit anywhere
Without realization of a missed place hair
The issue has gone
Tweet, Tweet. Tweet,
Replaced by a cheerful bird song

EASTER 2002

March arrived with Edward cutting everyone out of his life, he appeared briefly when Dan or Holly were around just to show his face, but always returned to his room after a few moments. His CPN called in to see him once at the request of Dan, but he said she stayed about ten minutes and Edward was able to hold it together for that amount of time, though his eye contact was poor. Every time I managed to get him on the phone he spoke in a black American rapper voice, he would never see me if I called round to the house, we spoke with a closed door between us. I phoned his CPN, which took courage on my part because I really felt she did not like me, and did not wish to communicate with me about my son. She was her cold self and seemed to take delight in making me feel small, she claimed she had seen him recently and he was fine. (Of course he was, he was going to get a job in McDonalds.)

I asked her "Is he still talking like a black rapper?"

She said "He did have a strange accent but he is into rap music, as are a lot of young people his age."

I said "I know that, but I felt he really thought he was a rapper."

She didn't think so "He may be a little delusional, but it's nothing to worry about, he's fine." End of phone call.

At another time when I spoke to Dan about our joint worry over Edward, he said he didn't think Edward was taking his medication, and I reminded him that Edward had told me he hadn't taken any since he left hospital in September last year. Dan said he was due to remind Edward he required a repeat prescription. I said what if you don't remind him and wait until he asks you, we'd know then if he was taking his medication. Dan said he would have to ask permission from his CPN but he thought it might be a good way of finding out if Edward really was taking his medication or not. His new CPN refused to allow that, and used my suggestion against me at the inquest; she made it look as if I was plotting against my son for some reason. Dan was so worried he phoned Paramount Housing the people he worked for who ran the Sheltered Homes to gain permission to go into his room to check on his medication and see if he was storing it. He was given permission but unfortunately Edward caught him going into his room, and he was not only unable to check, but it made Edward lose some of his trust in Dan.

The second week in March and my daughters Birthday, we had arranged as a family to go out for a meal. I spoke to Dan about Edward coming and he felt it would be too stressful for him to be out in public for an evening. He was finding it hard being in the house with others and spent a lot of time in his room. When I tried to phone him he would not come to the phone. The following weekend was my mothers eightieth Birthday and my sister who lives near her in Essex was arranging a party, again I could not reach Edward, or see him when I called. I talked constantly with Dan at this time as we were both worried and not sure what we could do. I spent the weekend in Essex and on my return tried to phone Edward, again he would not come to the phone.

On the Thursday of that week Mourn Day Thursday I phoned again this time he picked up the phone, he was hostile and sharp and said, " No he did not want to join me over Easter." This worried me as I knew there would be no staff on duty, and most of the others would have gone home. I was really worried about his mental condition now and I phoned the Fair Mile to try and talk to his consultant. They took my number and said they would phone back, eventually Holly the care assistant of the house in Selsea Place called me back and just told me he was alright, spending most of his time in his room. She had seen him briefly; he was quite sharp in his speech, but always very polite. That's alright then, I thought as I put down the phone, as long as he's polite I don't have to worry!

Good Friday passed with me worrying about Edward's health and feeling helpless. How I could see him, when he refused any sort of contact. Easter Saturday I tried to make the best of things and set about getting things ready for Easter Sunday, and family coming for lunch. But Ed' was always at the back of my mind. Then at about four thirty Saturday afternoon Edward rang me, and asked if he could come over for the Easter.

Delighted at his change of mind Nick and I went to collect him. He was ready and waiting when we arrived at the house, and came out with his weekend bag. He seemed very calm, and not as restless as he usually was when becoming unwell, he looked awful, very pale all most grey, the area around his eyes was dark and his eyes very sunken. He took his bag up to his room and sat and watched television, always when he was unwell, he would sit very close to the screen and become so engrossed I use to have to touch him, to make him aware I was trying to talk to him. I made his favourite supper that evening, he ate most of it, he seemed very quiet and thoughtful. After supper we decided to watch the video "What a Woman Wants" with Mel Gibson, a light-hearted comedy. About half way through the film Edward left the room, I thought he'd gone out for a cigarette.

When he didn't return I went out to see if he was alright, he was at the desk where the computer was and busy writing. When he saw me he quickly folded up the papers and stuffed them in his pocket. I apologized for disturbing him and thought he was writing poetry or rap songs. Nick went up to bed after the film, and Ed' and I talked for awhile about the family, he asked how his sister and brother were and I filled him in, and reminded him he would be seeing them on Sunday, along with Nicks son and family.

At eleven he went up to bed to listen to a rap programme he liked, a few moments later he came down and said his programme wasn't on, that they were playing classical music. I said I thought it was because the Queen Mother had died, and he stayed down stairs with me and we talked about music. When we went up to bed he turned to me and said "I love you mum." and I replied "I love you to Ed' and we went into our rooms. He was very restless and I could hear him moving about for sometime, but I eventually fell asleep.

At about two thirty that morning I awoke to a loud pounding on the bedroom door. Edward burst in the passage light was on and he stood in the door way with the light behind him. He had his jeans on and no top, the front of his chest was covered with blood, there was a gap hanging from the left side of his neck, and a red line right across his throat area running with blood.

He said "Mum I've tried to kill myself I've cut my throat."

I was already pulling on my dressing gown by this time I said something like "Oh, my God, Edward!" As I moved past him he handed me the papers he had stuffed into his pocket earlier, this turned out to be his suicide note, this I did not read until sometime later. I ran down stairs to the phone I was shaking and unable to think straight. I called the Fair Mile that was the hospital where Edward was a patient so I thought they were the right people to contact. They told me to phone his GP's surgery.

"No doctor would be on duty at 2-30 a.m. on Easter Sunday" I yelled down the phone.

Nick by now had come too and realized what had happened, he was with Edward and he called down the stairs, "Phone a fucking ambulance."

This I did and then rushed to pull on some clothes,

in the bathroom I saw one of my kitchen knives and a lot of blood in the hand basin. I realized Edward had stood in front of the mirror to watch what he was doing. Nick cleaned this while I was away at the hospital.

Nick waited outside for the ambulance, and I sat with Edward, he'd tried to wipe the blood from his chest and had pulled on a sweat shirt. He now sat in an armchair holding a new three corner bandage against his neck, the thickest thing I could find in the first aid box. I knelt on the floor holding his free hand and trying to comfort him. While we waited he told me, he had been thinking he was a famous rapper, and that he had had an affair with Foxy Brown another rappers wife. All the rappers had found out about this and three men from London were coming down to kill him in a slow and terrifying way. He was being told that it would be better if he killed himself. He said he had heard the men outside the house and that was what had driven him to cutting his throat.

He kept saying "Mum I don't want to die, I'm really scared." I told him I didn't want him to die and that he was very ill and needed to be in hospital. He agreed and said "I know I'm mentally ill, but this is all very real to me." I said I understood, and that was why it was very important to get medical help.

The paramedics arrived and asked Nick if it was safe to enter the house, he assured them it was. They were very good with him when they saw the state of his neck they said they would have to take him to hospital. I travelled with him and left Nick to phone Edward's father. At the hospital we were taken into a cubical and Edward lay on the bed I sat on the only chair. I waited until a nurse assessed the injury, and I explained Edward's mental condition to her. She said he would need sutures and she would contact the duty psychiatrist to come and asses him as well. She stayed with him while I went outside to phone Nick and tell him what was happening, and spoke to my daughter and other son. The whole time Edward was in the John Radcliff he was never once left alone. Adrian eventually arrived just before the doctor came in to attend Edward. He had internal and external sutures. The doctor explained to Edward he had used dissolving sutures and that he had done it in such a way that when the wound had healed, no one would ever know what he had done; it would look like a crease in his neck. Edward was pleased about that and thanked the doctor. The doctor then put some steri-stitches over the sutures to help hold things in place.

The doctor said to Edward that he noticed he seemed very agitated and he felt concerned for him. Edward explained that three men were out to kill him and that they were outside the hospital, that he could sense they were trying to come in and find him. The doctor told him he didn't have to see anyone unless he wanted to, that he would send them away, if Edward said that was what he wanted. This seemed to calm Edward for awhile.

We waited for several hours for the duty psychiatrist to appear, but they had a more urgent case, and eventually we were shown into the Barnes Unit an over night ward for people who had attempted harm to themselves during the night. Edward had a bed, Adrian sat on the end of it and I sat on the floor for what proved to be a very long wait.

Some time in the morning Jane arrived and sat with us, Edward at one point went and had a wash, shave, and cleaned his teeth. On his return one of the steri-stitches had come adrift and a little blood was seeping out. Edward was concerned about it, a nurse looked at it for him, and reassured him it was all right as the sutures were still in place. She then asked if he had his medication on him, he said yes and she gave him some water to take it. I know he took it the night before because I had insisted he took it while I watched, and the nurse watched him in the morning.

At around twelve that morning the duty psychiatrist called us into a room, I told her of Edward's illness and what had happened, and then she had a long talk to Edward. He explained his fears and told her all he had told me.

He finished with "I'm really scared I don't want to die."

The doctor said she understood this, and said "What if I told you no men are coming to kill you?"

Edward replied, "I know that's what you think and my mum and family, I know I'm mentally sick, but it's very real to me, and I'm really scared I don't want to die."

The doctor said she understood how real it was to him, and that she agreed he was mentally ill and he needed to be in hospital, that she would see if she could find him a place. I told her his consultant came from the Fair Mile, but he was away for the Easter break. I wish now I had not said anything and let her find a hospital; my son would still be alive if he hadn't gone to the Fair Mile. At the time I thought I was doing the right thing. We were with that doctor for an hour; she said she would phone the Fair Mile and fax all the information including a copy of the suicide note I had shown her.

We waited another hour and she came and apologized, she said she had spoken to the duty doctor at the Fair Mile an hour ago and he said he would get back to her in ten minutes, and she was still waiting, that she was going to try again. She then directed us to the hospital canteen. Edward came with us he had an orange juice, but did not want to eat, we had a sandwich each and a drink, but I was too wound up to eat all of mine.

We waited another hour and the doctor came to us again, She apologized, and said the Fair Mile doctor had not rang back since her second call. "I'm going to phone again and see if I can get a positive reply."

She came back about half an hour later, said she had spoken to the duty doctor, that the Fair Mile had a bed. She had faxed all the information over to the doctor and they were expecting us. We were to take him to Ibsden Ward; we thanked her and made our way to the cars. I travelled with Adrian and Edward, Jane followed in her car. As we passed Tesco's Edward asked if we could stop to buy him a sandwich, I had to explain it was Easter Sunday and it was the one day that shops closed including Tesco. I said it was half an hour to four O'clock and I thought the hospital would be having tea soon.

At the Fair Mile we reported to the reception desk and were given instructions on how to reach Ibsden ward. The hospital was dark and dismal, an old Victorian Institution, it was due to close the following year and it looked very neglected, but I thought the people in the hospital would remain professional and caring to the last moment for the sake of the patients in their care. We walked through several corridors and doors up stairs and even more corridors until we at last reached the Ward.

When we entered the place seemed chaotic, unorganized, and grubby, people were wondering around aimlessly it was difficult to say who was a patient and who was a nurse. To me they all looked like patients as they all stared at us, but no one asked what we wanted. There was no notice to say where new patients should check in, nothing to say where the nurse's station was. I walked further into the large room towards a place that seemed to be full of hall like chairs in rows facing a television. I turned back towards the centre of the room or hall way, one of the people I'd seen earlier was a man in a safari suit holding a clip board, there was nothing to say who he was but I had to approach someone. I asked him where I could find a nurse, he made no reply but led me to a small room farther along, and there a nurse greeted Edward and the rest of us. She said the doctor was on another ward and showed us into a tiny room with book shelves, she asked us to wait and she would phone the doctor, that he would be with us in a few minutes.

I sat opposite Edward, Jane on the same side as me and Adrian near to Edward, the window was open it had been a nice day but it was the last day of March and the warmth had left the sun by evening and it was getting cold. After a moment I shut the window, it was a scruffy little room, half eaten sandwich was drying on one of the book shelves. Clothes were scattered on some of the seats, milk left on top of the fridge and several dirty cups seemed to be the main décor to the place. The nurse put her head around the door twice to apologize for the doctor keeping us waiting. Above Edwards head was a wall clock and I watched the time tick round to four thirty.

Just after four thirty the doctor arrived, he came into the room like a crusader, with a great flourish he sat between Edward and Adrian, the doctor was followed by the man in the safari suit and clip board. The doctor told us his name Dr. Mason; he did not introduce the other person who followed him in. He asked us what had been going on, Edward explained his fears about three men coming from London, who were going to torture him to death. That they were telling him it would be better to kill himself, before they caught him. He explained on March 27th he had come to realise he was mentally ill. He explained the voices were very real to him.

Dr. Mason then asked him how he felt. I remember Edward's exact words because he'd been saying it all day.

"I'm scared shitless, I don't want to die."
Dr. Mason then asked if he had a gun would he use it. Edward looked surprised by the question and he replied,

"Where would I get a gun and why would I want to shoot anyone?"

We went onto the events that happened earlier that day, when Edward had cut his throat. I explained what had happened and our time spent at the John Radcliff and the treatment he had received. I offered Dr. Mason Edward's suicide note that I had in my bag. He declined to look at it saying,

"That's the one with the joined up writing faxed from the J.R." to me it sounded like he thought Edward not capable of writing in such a way. Dr. Mason continued with the fact that Edward's consultant was away until Tuesday. That they would keep Edward on Ibsden until then. He then said to me,

"You say he did this injury to his neck early yesterday morning?" I explained that it had happened at 2-30 a.m. this morning.

Dr. Mason said "So you guys have had no sleep." We agreed we hadn't he then turned to Edward "Don't you think you have put these guys through enough. I think they should go home." I said I wanted to stay until Edward was settled in.

Dr Mason turned to Edward again, "You don't need your mother here do you. These guys have had no sleep."

I felt we were being dismissed and Edward was being made to feel guilty. Edward made no reply but I could see he was becoming stressed. I assured Edward I would be in to see him the next day if we had to leave now.

Dr. Mason turned to Edward "You don't need your mother to visit tomorrow. You can give her a day off can't you?"

Edward was now upset and said "I do want to see mum in the morning." I assured him I would be there and so did his father.

Dr. Mason then explained that Edward would be moved on Tuesday to his consultants ward and that there was a small possibility that Edward would have to be moved to another hospital. This really alarmed Edward and worried me. We asked " Why?"

He did not give a reason, but just replied "It is only a remote possibility." Then he walked out followed by the other person. My daughter thought he said something as he left, But I did not hear him say anything. We sat not sure what to do, discussing whether we were able to stay or were we meant to go. Edward was very agitated and suddenly left the room and went into the corridor. I followed him out and saw the man with the clip board. "What are we to do, are we meant to go or can we stay?" I asked.

"You can go." were his only words.

I walked over to Edward and the others and told them we were to go, I hugged and kissed Edward told him I loved him and would be in to see him first thing in the morning. The others made their farewells and we walked to the door, there I turned back to look at him. He stood with his bag over one shoulder; he looked near to tears and lost like a small boy. I wanted to say "It's alright Edward come back with me I'll look after you." But I didn't say a word; logic told me I was leaving him in a place of safety. A place where professionals would care for him and give him the correct medication and help make him feel better, I just waved and went through the door. I did not realize that was the very last time I would see my son conscious, and the very last time we would hug each other.

We made our way out through the maze of corridors, doors and stairs to our cars. I was to travel back with Jane, Adrian lived in the other direction from us, we spoke for a while about what had happened, and all three of us were relieved that he was now safe. On the journey back I began to relax and realized how tired I was, I also kept thinking of him pulling the knife across his throat and kept shaking at the thought. I arrived home at five- thirty, I only know this because Nick had just looked at the time before I arrived. He was becoming worried I'd been out of the house since three thirty that morning.

Nick hugged me as I filled him in on the day's events, I told him I didn't like the doctor who had interviewed Edward at the Fair Mile I said I found him arrogant, and told him about the odd questions he asked and how he reacted towards us. Nick thought maybe he was just concerned about what we had been through. I said that was probably right, but I wished he had not made Edward feel guilty about it. I felt that was wrong, I wished he had shown more compassion towards my son his patient rather than his family, who would recover from lack of sleep.

Nick had prepared a meal, but suggested a drink at our local pub to relax me before we ate. I went across with him and we had a couple of drinks and chatted to several people, I was on a high now, the crisis with my son was over and I could let go for awhile and let others take the responsibility. On our return the message button on the phone was flashing, it was Adrian asking me to call him. I felt a terrible feeling of foreboding as I rang him, he said he had called the hospital at six to ask if Edward had settled in, the person he spoke to said they would go and look, they came back to say they could not find him. Adrian then drove over to the Fair Mile and made his way up to the Ward. This time the door was locked and he had a problem getting in, eventually they opened the door. They said they had searched the ward and the grounds that someone had gone to his flat as he had at one point asked to go home. They had staff out looking round the area and the police had been informed, they were going to bring out the police helicopter if he wasn't found soon. He told me he had been out searching and that Jake and his fiancée were also out searching, for me to stay were I was in case Ed' was making his way back to Blewbury.

I put the phone down with shaking hands, my whole world seemed to have stopped, and I felt as if I was suspended in some sort of nightmare. I couldn't eat or sit still I was trembling and restless. Around nine O' clock the phone rang again it was Adrian, he was at the Fair Mile and so were the police, they had had a call from the transport police from

Reading station, they said a youth had fallen from the top of the station car-park and was being taken to the Royal Berkshire Hospital in Reading. We did not know if it was Edward but Adrian was going to make his way to the hospital. I called Jack on his mobile and asked if he could pick Nick and me up. He explained he was already half way to Reading, so I said I'd see him there. I rang Adrian back and asked him if we could travel with him. He agreed to collect us and while we waited I phoned Jane, like me she felt before she answered the phone that it was to be bad news. She followed us in her car to the hospital.

All the way there we kept talking about what had happened, not believing that Edward had left
the hospital unnoticed. We were convinced the person at the Royal Berks. was not Edward, but we felt we had to check to make sure. As the person had no identification on them, no one knew who he was, so we at least could help the police rule out it being Edward. It would have only taken one of us to go, but we were all up tight and very restless, we had a need to be doing something. The police and staff were still searching for Edward, and we needed to be involved in some way, eliminating the person at the Royal Berks. seemed to be something we could do.

When we arrived at the A&E I went up to the reception as soon as we said our name a nurse came to us, we were shown into a restricted area and from there to a small family room. Jack and

Louise were already there they were both in tears.

“It is Ed’ mum,” Jack sobbed “they have just asked if he had a recent injury to his neck.” As I hugged and tried to comfort them both I felt my heart sink and tears burn the back of my eyes. Jack said they had now stabilized him and that he was being taken for a scan. I sat on one of the plastic chairs and stared at the wall opposite, where a poster seemed to mock me. It was larger than A3 size and it explained that mental illness could affect most families at some time. It gave various things to look out for and that one in four took their own lives, it pleaded with relative and friends to seek help before it was too late. I kept reading it over and over again and anger bubbled up inside me. In the end I ripped the poster off the wall and put it into my bag. Several days later I wrote in black marker pen in large upper case, “**Edward’s family were there, we did not leave it too late, where were you**?” and I sent it to Ibsden ward.
I just wish I had been there when they opened it.

It seemed some time before a doctor came to us, but I had lost all sense of time, very little registered except for news of my youngest son. The doctor introduced himself and sat on a seat looking at us all he was very sombre and I knew the news was not going to be good.
He said “ You're son was conscious when he was brought in, he tried to speak, but due to a broken jaw and other facial injuries we could not understand him, we had to sedate him as soon as

we could. I'm afraid he is ninety- five percent close to death; he is hurt from the top of his head to the bottom of his feet. We need to operate to see to the internal injuries, before we take him up to the theatre you may come and see him very briefly, two at a time. I must warn you he fell face down and his injuries to his face are extensive."

Adrian and I followed him; he led us around a curtained cubical, not far from the little room we were in. What I saw took my breath away; I groaned his name as I took the sight of him in. His head was huge; I never realized a person could swell up so much. He looked like some horrific science fiction monster; his nose had been pushed to the side of his face all his features were hugely enlarged, blood came out of his nose, eyes, ears and mouth. I was so shocked all I could do was say his name over and over again, as tears ran down my face. The one thing that I saw that convinced me it was my son was a scar on his shoulder from a dog bite when he was seven. Adrian and I left as Jack and Louise were shown in. Nick put his arms around me as I sobbed "I've lost him." Nick went in with Jane by the time they came out we were all in tears and comforting each other. I couldn't believe all this was happening and I was finding it hard to realize it was real. It all seemed like some horrendous dream.

A nurse took us up to the intensive care area and showed us into a family room, there were two beds and a couple of chairs, there was also a place to make a hot drink, and a fridge of food and a microwave, and a bathroom. We never had any of the food, but Adrian had a need to be busy and made several cups of tea and coffee for everyone over the time we stayed there. I lay on one of the beds with Jane, Jack lay on the other and others took it in turn to lay on the beds and use the chairs, none of us slept.

At one time in the night the doctor we had seen earlier came into us, I noticed blood on his operating clothes and knew it was Edward's. He said Edward had ruptured his liver and stomach and that they were having trouble stopping his liver bleeding. That blood was seeping out of his body all the time, but they were doing all they could to stop it. He said again how close Edward was to death.

He returned to the theatre and the next time he saw us, he said they had had to pack his liver and hoped that would stem the blood flow. That he was on a blood pressure machine to try and keep his blood pressure up, and said again that he was very near to death. He explained he had done all he could and that the surgeons that set broken bones were now going in.

I found myself crying again after the doctor left and feeling very low, I didn't think I could bare it if he died, and I said prayers in my head and pleaded silently to God, for him to live. When the next surgeon came to us he seemed very positive and for a while we felt uplifted, he had set broken elbows, a foot on one leg, the ankle on the other, and his jaw. It took some while after he had gone to realize he was only being positive about his bones, but we were so desperate to hear something good that we clung to this news for some time, and felt a little better for a while. The next and last team to go in were the plastic surgeons after they had done all they could, they came to see us and said that he would need more operations once the swelling had gone down.

Then the first doctor we saw then came back in and said Edward had needed forty pints of blood, and that the blood pressure machine was having trouble keeping his blood pressure up, that he was now in Intensive Care and we could go and see him when ever we wanted to.

Intensive Care seemed to be a large room with beds around the nurse station in a semi-circle. Curtains were between the beds it was dark when I first went in with mooted light, making people at various beds staying by their loved ones look ghost like. The swelling of Edward's head if anything looked worse, I couldn't understand how his skin could stretch so far over the vast head, his nose was now in the correct place. There were various machines around him making odd little noises, tubes ran from under the bed clothes into containers on the floor, and I thought of blood seeping out of his body. I found it hard to stay with him for too long as I would start to sob and I didn't know if he could hear me, and I didn't want to worry him.

I had no idea how long he would be in Intensive Care I imagined it would be for several days if not weeks. I had not washed since my shower on Saturday or changed my cloths since the early hours of Sunday morning. Now dawn was breaking on Easter Monday morning, I spoke to a nurse and she said the doctors would be doing their rounds at around nine in the morning, I said I needed to go home and collect my wash things. She said it was a good time to go as Edward had only just come out of theatre and would not be coming round yet.

Jane took Nick and I home, she only lived four miles from us, and she returned to her home for fresh clothes and wash things. I had a quick shower changed my clothes and packed a bag to return to the hospital. Nick was to stay at home and contact other members of our families to tell them what had happened in the morning, dawn had only just broken. While I waited for Jane I phoned the Wallingford Mental Health Team and left a message on their answer phone for the stuck up CPN I told her she may have read the books and taken the exams, but she needed to listen to members of her patient's families and friends as they knew the person, she didn't. I filled her in on what had happened and told her my son was likely to die. She never ever contacted me, not even after Edward died to give her condolences, and she again snubbed me at the inquest. I often wonder what a person like that was doing in mental health when they had no empathy or compassion.

It was very surreal driving back to the hospital with Jane, it was Easter Monday the sun was shinning and a few people were just beginning to appear. There was little traffic, some shops were beginning to open, and all around the world seemed to be carrying on as normal. I felt as if I was in some sort of plastic bubble, where only pain and tears existed, it was as if Jane and I were in some sort of time warp, everything seemed slow moving and silent when I now think back. We hardly spoke on the return journey, both deep in thought of our own fears.

As soon as I arrived back at the hospital I went into to see Edward, there was a group of people around him, an older doctor came up to me, and asked if I was his mother. He told me Edward had had a terrible trauma to his whole body and that if he managed to survive the body trauma, there was still brain damage to consider. He said they had been unable to drill holes to relieve the pressure to his brain due to the injuries to his skull, and that I should prepare myself for the worse. I think I thanked him and went back to the little family room, but I don't really remember how I got back to the room; I felt by then that all hope had left me. My youngest child was just clinging on to life, and there was nothing I could do to help him live.

Jane and Adrian were not in the room when I

returned; Louise and Jack looked pale and exhausted. A nurse came in and said the police would like a word with me. Jack came with me there were two detectives who asked about Edward and what had happened. I filled them in with all I knew and Jack told them other things. They asked me a couple of time if there was anything I wanted them to do. I couldn't think clearly and did not really know what they wanted me to say. I just said please find out what went wrong and why Edward was allowed to leave a hospital that was suppose to keep him safe. I realize now they probably wanted me to ask them to find out who was responsible. But my mind was numb to everything but the pain and fear I felt for my son.

I kept going in to see Edward, and leaving as I became too upset, not wanting to let Edward hear me, or disturb other patients and troubled relatives. Mid morning a nurse asked us all to go into the doctor's room that was part of the Intensive Care Unit. As we followed the nurse I said "This is not going to be good news."

Adrian replied "You don't know that, it may be good."

In the office were several chairs for us to sit on, a light box was on and the scan of a head was pinned on it. I knew it had to be Edward's scan, though Adrian said it may not be, I felt they would not leave a scan of someone else lit up for us to see. When the doctor came in I could see he was very upset, it was the same doctor we had first met in the trauma unit, and had fought all night in the theatre to save him.

He explained that Edward's brain had swollen, and that it would continue to swell for the next seventy-two hours, that it had coned (meaning it had seeped down into his neck) He showed us on the scan, and also pointed out how Edwards face had been pushed over to one side of his head, he pointed out the swelling of his brain and said the stem of the brain could not be seen due to the swelling. He told us the blood pressure machine could not keep his blood pressure up. He said if he did manage to survive the terrible trauma to his body, he would be in a complete vegetable state. He asked us to consider turning of the life support machines. He was really upset and explained how they hated giving up on one so young, but there was nothing else they could do to help him.
We were all crying. I sat between Jane and Jack and we had our arms around each other as we wept, Louise sat next to Jack crying and holding him. Adrian was unable to accept what the doctor said at first, and walked around pleading and begging him to find some way of saving Edward, as he wept.

Eventually Adrian accepted what the doctor said, and we hugged each other and talked it over through our tears. We knew we had no choice, but it was the hardest and worse thing any of us has ever had to do. Even though we knew it was only machines that were keeping him going, none of us wanted to let Edward go, but in the end we had to do the right thing for Edward, however much pain it gave us.

I had always thought that you literally just turned off a machine and the person died, the way it's portrayed in films, but that was not how it was with Edward. I had a chair near to him, and I stroked his arm just above the plaster to his elbow, his hands were under the covers across his middle. Adrian stood at his head, Jack opposite me, Jane by my side, and dear Louise upset and tearful as she was, went from one to the other of Edward's family hugging us and supporting us, she was only a young girl in her twenty's, but she was amazing that Easter Monday. A nurse came in the curtained area around us every so often and did things to the various machines, and slowly reduced the sedation being administered to him.

Jack kept pleading with him not to die and said over and over how he loved him, Jane cried quietly by my side telling him she loved him, Adrian stroked his hair on his over enlarged forehead, his hair stiff and red coloured with dried blood, tears running down his face. I kept telling Edward how much I loved him, and how proud I was of him, I told him I was there with him. Every so often I would be over come with heavy sobbing, and I'd lay my head by his side as I wept uncontrollably and beg him to stay with us.

Around lunch time a nurse put her head around the curtain and said there was someone on the phone from the Fair Mile, they were asking after Edward, and she could not tell them anything due to confidentiality, I said I would speak to them. I introduced myself, it was a staff nurse from Ibsden Ward, I told her Edward was dieing, and she said how sorry she was. Something inside me snapped and I said, “He shouldn’t be here, he should be safe with you that‘s where I left him, why isn’t he still safe with you?”

She replied “We inadvertently misplaced him.” Her words to me, made him sound like a package rather than a human being, and I felt anger, I don’t recall what else I said if anything. I didn’t want to talk to her any more and I know I ended the call when I heard beeping coming from where Edward was, I needed to go back to him. I ended the call with”I have to get back to my dieing son,” and put down the phone. I did not give the call another thought, though now I realize it must have been distressing for the staff nurse. But my mind at that time could only grasp what was happening to my youngest child, I could not think or feel anything else.

Louise went out to phone Nick to let him know what was happening, and he was soon sitting with us. Our eyes kept being drawn to the heart monitor, we just couldn’t help it, even after Nick, who had already been through what we were going through with his wife, advised us to keep looking at Edward, that the machine meant nothing. He told us the machine would slow down then would quicken up and then slow down very rapidly as the end came. A nurse came in at one point and took a cover off Edward as she said he was getting too hot, the heart monitor went crazy for a moment as he reacted to the removal of the cover. This gave me a tiny glimmer of hope, because I had seen a small response, all the time I was looking for signs that the medical team were wrong, yet deep down I knew there was no hope, I only had to look at that awful grotesque head to know the real truth. The nurse also removed his hands from under the covers, and I took hold of one and held it between both of mine, Jack held the other hand. Now when I look back I can only see that hand as being small and delicately child like, against mine, due to his head being so out of proportion to the rest of his body. I find it impossible to recall his hands as being as big if not bigger than mine, yet they were as he was a six foot twenty year old man.

Adrian kept wiping away blood from his face with a tissue, so the nurse brought in a small bowl and some cotton wool so we could wash him. Jane and I washed his hands that were covered in dried blood. Jack and Adrian carefully washed his face, it was so dark with bruises that in the end I became worried they were hurting him, and I had to ask them to stop. The whole time this was happening we were tearful, odd moments we remembered things about Edward and we spoke of them, the odd smile came between our tears. Due to Edward being religious during his illness when we were asked if we wanted someone from the church to see Edward, we said yes, prayers were said for him and he was blessed.

Middle afternoon the heart machine began to slow down, I remembered Nick's words, and my heart that had been racing since Edward had cut his neck, began to pound in my chest, and I begged Edward not to leave us. True to Nicks prediction the monitor began to show rapid heart beats, and then it slowed very quickly until it stopped, at three twenty-four on first of April 2002 my youngest son died. I was completely stricken with pain and tears I lay across Edward crying for him to come back, the worse thing I could ever imagined had just happened, and I was going to have to bare it the same as everyone did, that went through the loss of a child. It is such a hard thing to bear, seeing a child you have loved and nurtured die. We were all in tears, and a nurse suggested we went out for a moment while they removed all the tubes and machines and then we could come back and sit with him.

We huddled together in tears in the doctor's office until we could return to Edward. I don't know how long we sat with Edward, most of what happened after his death seemed to be in a fog for the rest of that day. At one point I remembered Edward carried a Dona-card and that he and I had spoke of it several times. I mentioned it to a nurse and someone appeared with a form. Adrian and I were asked a lot of question everything seemed to go well, until they asked if he had ever injected drugs. Though I doubted that he ever did due to his fear of injections I could not say for certain that he hadn't, and neither could Adrian so that was the end of that. I felt disappointed because I knew Edward had felt very strongly about being a Dona. When we were ready to leave Edward and go home, we were taken downstairs and asked to wait in another small room. A nurse came in with various leaflets, which she handed to Adrian and me. We were told there would be an inquest and a post mortem as it was an unexpected death, and that we would have to return the following day to formally identify the body?

Stunned we left the hospital brought some flowers, scribbled messages on odd scraps of paper we found in the car and attached them to the flowers. We made our way to Reading Station Multi-Story Car-Park, found the signs where Edward had actually fell and left the flowers on the spot. We then made our way up to the top floor and looked down to the spot where he fell and must have stood before it happened. The police that morning said they had found a packet of sandwiches, an orange juice and his cigarettes on the wall where he had left them. I have not been able to visit the station or the car-park since that day.

SOME ANGELS

Send me down some Angels,
So I can amend what is unfixed,
One piece for me, save my sanity
To secure a mind deeply lost in despair
And set it back on a path of thoughtfulness.

Some Angels for nature, a poor dying breed,
So nature can breathe easy, before suffocation
Flourishes after fulfilling its need.
A piece for the atmosphere we pollute
We foolishly, knowingly, aid our own death.

Some Angels for love, for now greed conquers all.
Unconsciously we are taken prisoner
Like crops infested with locus
We cry I want, I will, I need. Success.
Always success with no love at all.

Some Angels for the poor, sick, and needy,
Those abandoned, alone no where to go.
Our ignorance pretends not to see, blind?
As we sit cold hearted at home with no wisdom,
Give respect, what would it cost?

Some Angels for peace, weapons needed to protect,
And war and killing we use as solutions.
Angels for peace, but the governments…I doubt?
As society kills another child, tears of loss.
Let harmony and negotiation reign supreme

Some Angels for children born into this world.
Send down some Angels, plus one for me.
If I don't ask for it to be done, who will?
One piece for me and my sanity
To secure a mind deeply lost in despair.

AFTER EDWARD'S DEATH

We all went back to Blewbury after we left Reading, we sat in the kitchen drinking tea, I and Jack went up into the attic looking through Edward's things, and we brought down some of his books, sketch pads and writings. We discovered he kept a diary from the age of nine to twelve the entries became more spasmodic as he grew older. Jack and I read parts out to everyone. A lot of the entries were very funny and we found ourselves laughing at times. The words brought Edward back to us and for a while and briefly we pushed aside the terrible tragic loss of life. As his words brought the old happy cheerful boy back into our lives. I found things of Edward's for Jane, Jack and Adrian to take home. Before they left Adrian, Nick and I arranged to meet up in the morning to return to the hospital.

The following morning Jane asked to come with us. I spoke to my mother several times on the phone just after Edward's death and I longed for her to be by my side, or at least my sister to be there, I had a terrible need for female company and my family. But neither came and I thanked God for Nick, without him I'm sure I could never have survived those first awful few weeks.

At the hospital we were directed to the Chapel of Rest where the Coroners Officer was waiting for us. He asked us what had happened and we told him about Edward falling from the Station Car Park and what happened after. He then asked us to formally identify Edward and he opened the door to the Chapel. Edward was laying in a coffin on a deep blue cloth, his huge face turned towards us. I could only go to the door I could not go into the Chapel. Adrian went into the Chapel and sat down, we confirmed it was Edward and the Coroner said he would wait outside and give us some time with Edward. Adrian and then Jane spent some time with Edward in the Chapel with the door closed, but I could not bring myself to go in, I couldn't bare to look at his poor broken body, and Edward was not there any more, to me it was just the shell that housed the person called Edward, his spirit had left.

Nick said he though we should have told the Coroners Officer about the cut throat and the "Cock up of the Fair Mile." He went outside to talk to the Officer, they both came back and the Officer asked us in more detail what had happened over Easter. He was really shocked when he heard the events that happened before his death, and explained we could not do the inquest by ourselves as it was not a straight forward death, that we would need a solicitor, as he was sure the Fair Mile would be arranging for a good solicitor for themselves. He said someone should be made responsible for what happened, and he had a lot of empathy for us. This man proved to be a tremendous support to me over the coming months; he kept in touch with me, constantly encouraging me to find a solicitor. Once I found one he kept me up to date with what was happening, and advised me all the way to the Inquest, that was not held until seven months after Edward's death. It was cancelled twice due to the hold up of Dr. Mason delaying in giving his statement. He also cut a lock of Edwards's hair for me that I keep in a gold locket.

After Easter the builders were to start the extension, several bits of building equipment had already been delivered; Nick rang them and put the start date off for two weeks. Adrian and I set about arranging the funeral, and hundreds of cards, and flowers started to arrive. I have no idea how so many people found out, I was amazed at the kindness of people, and some were people I had lost touch with over the years. My sitting room began to look like a florist, the most touching thing were three letters from Edwards friends he had known since the age of nine, they are so special. Nick advised me to have a box and put things I felt were close to Edward in it, this I did starting with his base ball cap and bandana, he had left at home when he was taken to hospital after his first attempt on his life that dreadful day. I can still smell him on them to this day. All the cards and the three letters are also in the box, I go through the box from time to time and certain things bring back treasured memories.

I was numb for a very long time, after Edwards's death, that is not to say I didn't cry because I did, I cried until I could not cry any more, and my body ached from the tears. The numbness was not being able to feel other things, it was like my feelings were blunt, I did things by automation or because that was what was expected of me. This strange blunt numb feeling lasted for a terribly long time; I did not even realize I felt like this until it started to lift.

Life just went on and I bobbed along like a cork in a vast sea. In reality all I wanted to do was stay in bed and sleep so I couldn't remember, but sleep rarely came and when it did it never lasted very long. Life had to go on, and my body kept breathing, so I carried on living. I drank more than usual around this time, but it had very little effect on me, and it did not ease the pain. The numbness was not there for the pain of Edward, I think that had taken me over so much; my body was in some way trying to protect me from other everyday stresses. Anything out of the ordinary happening and I would just go to pieces. The once very organized capable person, who battled with everything and took things in her stride, does not seem to be there any more, now I struggle to cope with every day life, though very few realize what's going on inside me, I put a face on for the world, but my world is not the same.

Edward's funeral was on the tenth of April 2002 a sunny windy day. Jane and I didn't wear black I felt he was young and black was too sombre. Edward was a lively fun loving person; he wouldn't have wanted people to wear black. I did request spring colours to be worn, so there was a mixture some in black others in lighter clothes. We had a family service at the crematorium where my mother, brother and his family, and my sister joined us, and Edward's other grandma. After that a service of celebration of Edwards's life was held at the local village Church where my three children had grown up. I had lived in the village of Ewelme for over thirty years, a lay preacher who had taught my older two children at the village school and knew Edward took part of the service, with the rector who also knew Edward. Both had been kind enough to visit me in Blewbury after Edwards's death and offered me comfort.

When I and the family walked into the Church that sunny April morning I could not believe how full it was, so many people. I read parts of Edwards's diary, Adrian read something about Edwards's life, and some of Edwards's poems were read. We played "Who Wants To Live For Ever" by Queen a favourite of both Jack and Edwards. We also played a song written and sung by Beth Nielson Chapman "No One Knows But You" the words to this song seemed to sum up all my feelings, even now when I think of Edward and start to miss him I have a need to play this song, often it reduces me to tears, but in an odd way it helps me too.
The first verse say's it all

“I can almost feel you smiling
From beyond those silver skies
As you watch me finding my way
Here without you in my life.
No one knows but you
How I feel inside”

When I stood at the door of the Church after the service I was really moved by so many people who attended, people whom I'd known years ago who had moved out of the village before me. Friends Edward had known since playgroup, and mothers I'd known from those days – many of his school friends from his prep school and all the teachers who had taught Edward. His house master from his last school whom I knew Edward liked and several friends from this school. Friends not from the village or school but whom we'd known since the early sixties, villagers and people I worked with. Dan came from Selsea Place Edward's last home with some of his house mates from Selsea Place. The social worker who gave me support when Edward was in limbo.

I was staggered and moved by so many people; we went down to the village hall where a couple of really good friends from Ewelme had laid on refreshments for everyone. It was a strange sort of day I walked from one group of people to another, not knowing what I said, I was in a daze. I didn't feel part of anything, and I couldn't grasp the fact that I had just seen my son in a closed coffin and that it was all over, that I'd never see him again. I wish now I could see many of those people and talk to them, especially Edwards's friends, all young men, looking older than their years on that day. Some had already been to a funeral the year before, for another friend from the school. Edward had been in hospital when Julian died I remember talking to him about it at the time, and how upset he had been. A few days after the funeral Harry, Edward's friend came and spent an afternoon with me, I really appreciated this visit and only wished I had been more aware of things, but at that time I seemed to be living in a permanent fog, though I found Harry's visit very comforting.

After the funeral we made our way back to Blewbury, Jane came with us and so did Jack and Louise, not wanting to go home we went over to the Barley Mow our local pub. We sat at a round table in the window with our drinks, when suddenly the Chef Andy came out with a large platter of warm finger food and put it into the middle of the table, and said it was on the house. I was really touched by this act of kindness, none of us had eaten that day and to sit in comfortable surroundings with people who knew where we'd been and were friendly and supportive, made an awful day seem a little better.

The odd simple acts of kindness shown to me by people over this time really helped me through those first few weeks. One couple that we did not know very well, a few days after Edwards's death

invited Nick and I round for a meal, neither of us had eaten much, and they gave us shepherds pie and rice pudding to follow, real comfort food. Friends just came up and hugged me, lost for words; others were straightforward and said "I don't know what to say to you." I appreciated all of them, the ones I found difficult to understand, were those who would cross over the street when they saw me, rather than acknowledge me, and the ones who would not let me talk, or said "aren't you over that yet", after only a few months.
Several days later I read a copy of Edward's suicide letter for the first time,

Dear mum dad Jack, Jane, Nick and family,
I'm really sorry but my mental illness must have gotten the better of me. I wish I stopped before I realized how serious it is, but it's too late. I love you all so much I wish it could be different, but I started thinking I was EminEm and I was Satan and I became obsessed with certain celebrities, I just wanted to make the world a better place, but I wish I realized sooner what I have done with my life. I know you've heard it all before but it looks like either I kill myself, or I'm going to be tortured and murdered as the things that were going on in my head must have got to the wrong people. I.E. rappers I became obsessed with. I became really confused and believed Foxy Brown was my wife and we loved each other and that I was EminEm. I don't know what to say just how sorry I am it had to be like this and it turned out like this. I love you so much and always will even though I won't be here

much longer. As I write this these people who want me dead for claiming to be the Messiah, masturbating etc are getting closer to finding me. I wish I had the bottle to talk to you about this, before they find me.

But I feel guilty messing my life up so much; I expect they will torture me to death. I believe they will and they will do their worse. I guess people just find out about things especially when you become mentally ill and get confused about some thing so serious. I suppose the wrong people find out and want me dead, because of it I wish they didn't but they do and it seems as though there's nothing I can do about it. I love you all so much, if there's a body to find, if there's anything left after they've finished with me, I'd like to be cremated. Please do what you want with the ashes if you want them, or want to do anything with them. I still got a feeling I was rapped whilst I slept in the mental hospital. I woke up with what looked like semen on my tea-shirt and I felt rapped in the morning and so did my body the way it moved etc. I believe it wasn't mental illness saying this, I was rapped. The rest though, about me being the Messiah wish I wasn't so stupid and realized before I got myself in all this trouble. I don't know what else to say except sorry, so sorry I didn't listen to you when you were just loving me and helping me. Guess you never expect this sort of thing is going to happen to you or in your case another family member. But it has happened it's too late and there's nothing nobody can do to change it. I love you so much, I'm sorry I always will love you all, love from Edward.

P.S. Just want to tell you I never rapped anyone ever, just masturbated too much, every day for weeks sometimes. And that I thought I was EminEm(tell you again just so you really know what I thought) EminEm with his body and face, Foxy Browns husband, I was Satan the devil who was Neo and my wife was Neon made of Electric and I was invisible and the Omen, I know I'm really ill but I was confused. I pray this won't happen to me the torture and murder but I fear and know it will. Love you loads Edward. Don't worry about me I'll be fine dead, please be happy for me, live the best possible life. And that when I realized on Friday 29th March how ill I was and how serious my condition was, how serious what I was saying and thinking it was too late to save my life. Miss you even though I'll be gone. It's Saturday 30th now I'm sitting at the desk whilst mum and Nick watch T.V. Miss you like crazy already even though I'll be dead and not there with you, always love you, your son, brother, friend love you forever Edward, sorry it had to end this way.

Even now May 2006 writing this and reading as I write tears run down my face, I can hear Edwards voice in my head saying the words, and I want so much to talk to him, to reassure him, to tell him there is no need to die, that we his family want him in our lives. But I never got the chance, I wish I had read it while we waited for the ambulance, after he had handed me the note, but at that time I was so concerned about him, I sat by his side holding his hand, the letter on the coffee table. I put it in my bag as we left for the hospital, so I could show the doctors; they made copies and faxed the pages onto the Fair Mile. On my return after leaving Edward at the Fair Mile I left it on the table still not reading it. At the time I thought it not relevant as the doctors were aware of its contents, and I believed he was now in a place of safety. Nick read it before me, while I was at the Royal Berks Hospital the following day, and it reduced him to tears.

Jack and Jane wanted a place to go to remember Edward, so we had his ashes interned in Ewelme graveyard. Where there is now a head stone and wild flowers have been planted round it. I could not go to the internment of the ashes, so soon after the funeral, I just couldn't bare it. The funeral directors gave me some of the ashes, and on Eve of New Year 2003 Nick and I scattered them around a bush that I call Ed in our garden. Fire works were lighting the sky, Church bells were ringing, and the horses in the field at the back of the garden were racing across the field, it was dark and very windy it seemed a magical moment as we stood with our arms around each other remembering him.

Just after Edward's death a good friend in Blewbury who use to be a psychiatric nurse told me to ask the Fair Mile for Edward's Observation Recording Sheet, she said this should have been written on each time someone checked on him. I phone for a copy straight away. It took them over two weeks to find it, they claimed his notes had gone missing, and they could not find them.

When the sheet eventually arrived I discovered he had only been on a fifteen minute watch and that they had his level of risk only at level three, level one being the highest risk of suicide, three the lowest, and that was after he had already attempted to kill himself earlier that day?. The sheet say's he was in the toilet at 16-45, on his bed at 17-00, at 17-15 asleep at 17-30 he was in the smoking room, at 17-45 he was missing. Then every fifteen minutes from that time it appears someone went to check on him and wrote missing all the way to 23-00 when the Royal Berkshire Hospital notified them. My friend told me they usually just wrote AWOL on the sheet at the time of the last check if someone was missing and then waited until the person showed up before continuing to write on the sheet.

It is only as I write all this four years later and reading all the notes and reports from the hospital at a time when I am rational and able to think clearly, that I note all the mistakes and cover up that went on after Edward's death.

Such as the fact that I know we were there until at least 17-00 he certainly did not have a bed at that time. At the inquest they claimed he also had dinner, but refused pudding, but that's not written on the Observation Sheet? Was he served his meal and did he eat it between the checks, a sick person with a painful neck/throat injury? There is so much evidence to suggest the people involved in Edward being able to walk out of the Fair Mile lied.

About a week after Edwards's death I had a need to go to his room in Selsea place, I had hoped to be by myself and sit and reflect on him for a while, but the whole family came with me, so I just started to collect his things and put them into black plastic bags. His room was the tidiest I had ever seen it apart from the day he had moved in. All his clothes were washed and folded in his drawers, all litter had been thrown out, and the floor vacuumed, he'd changed his bed-clothes, his dirty ones were in a neat pile on the floor. In his bedside drawer I found it to be full of medication, packets of them. If only Dan had had a chance to search his room that day he tried, or we had been allowed to see if Edward had asked for his repeat prescription at the correct time, rather than Dan having to remind him. Either of those things could have changed the events that happened. All Edwards's personal things were gone, apart from his radio and bible. There were no c.d's. none of his books, any note or sketch books, none of his odd bits of jewellery or his gold cross. Dan said he would ask the others in the house if he had given them away, and I said no if Edward had wanted them to have them, then that was fine, his wishes should be respected.

One really odd and not very pleasant thing happened in March 2003, I had a phone call from my solicitor to say the police had some of Edward's clothes did I want them.? Puzzled Nick and I went to Abingdon Police Station wandering as we travelled there, what clothes they were talking about, neither of us could figure it out. When we arrived at the police station we discover they were the clothes the paramedics had cut off of Edward at the scene.

The person on the front desk said “S.O.C.O. say’s they are covered with blood do you really want them?”

“No, get rid of them.” I almost screamed at her and we left the police station, I in tears and Nick devasted that we had been called out by the solicitor for that, when I phoned him to say what they were he seemed very detached and unconcerned, but the effect on me had been very disturbing.

DEATH

Speeding down the road as fast as I can
Whoops a daisy just run over a man
Red light
Green light
Catch me if you can
Better watch out for that van.
Pass my friend Mat.
Meow
Splat goes that cat.
Watch out for that old lady pushing a pram,
Oh look she just nicked some ham.
Slam on the brakes.
Bam goes the car.
Well I'll be damned
BLACK OUT
What a silly man!

WHAT HAPPENED NEXT

Not long after Edward's death his new consultant from the Fair Mile came to see me. I went through everything that had happened that weekend, and spoke in great detail about the interview with Dr. Mason. He advised me to write everything down while it was still fresh in my mind. He also said he hoped I was not going to just leave things as they are, that I deserve some answers, something needed to be done about my loss.
I took his advice and wrote down everything that had happened including times as I remembered

them. I had photos of Edward all around, because I could not get the last image of my son out of my head and I so desperately wanted to remember him without the terrible facial injuries.

The consultant said as he left "He was a good looking lad."

While the builders started the footings to the extension, I and Adrian went on a hunt for a solicitor. He found one in Wallingford who he'd used during our divorce, but what we needed was a medical solicitor. I contacted the N.S.F. co-coordinator in Oxford and she gave me several numbers to try, most I phoned were not able to help, but one in Oxford gave me an interview. I think she would have been helpful but at nearly £200.00 an hour there was no way I could afford her offer. I had to pay £50.00 just for the half an hour interview. After that I wrote half a dozen letters to solicitors in the yellow pages, who were no win no fee people. I Explained the circumstances and gave detail of what had happened. All wrote back to me, some saying it was not in their remit but wished me luck in finding a solicitor – one who had a branch in Blewbury replied with a positive out come, and I signed up with him. I had a long interview with him one hot May morning and told Edward's story. This turned out to be the first of many interviews over the next four and a half years. As with my letter it was the first of many hundreds I was to write, I had a very strong need to fight for Edwards's corner, to tell as many people as possible what had happened to my youngest child, and that "care in the community" did not work.

One of the first letters I wrote was a letter of complaint to the Royal Berkshire Mental Health Trust and also to the Fair Mile Hospital. I also wrote to Boris Johnson who had helped so much with Edward's benefits, he arranged to meet me to discuss what had happened, I was touched by his interest and met him in Thame one afternoon. I wrote to the Daily Mail, and they sent out a reporter and a photographer, but it was never used for some reason.

About a year after Edward's death a film company contacted me about Edward. They were making a series of documentaries about life changing events, called "Picking up the Pieces," for Channel 4. They were a young group and it was the directors first film, it all seemed to be done on a shoe string, and we received no payment, the reason why I and Jane put our selves through it was so more people could hear what had happened. My view to the whole thing was to try and stress the Berkshire Mental Health Trust, and to warn others of the dangers of thinking a loved relative would be in safe hands and cared for once in hospital, as it was not necessarily the case. They became closely involved with our lives for about nine months on and off, and then disappeared without a trace.

The Chief Nurse from the Royal Berkshire Mental Health Trust and a nurse from the Fair Mile came to see me. They said they were very sorry at what had happened, and that an internal inquiry was being carried out, that they would contact me when it was over and let me see the report. I was still numb and in shock it was difficult to think straight and ask the questions I would ask now. It was too soon for me to grasp anything properly, my hurt was so deep I could not express my pain to them. Sometimes I don't think many really know how bad this time has been and how much damage it has done to me. For them it is over now they've moved on, but part of me can never move on, I miss my son not being in my life.

With in a few weeks the shell of our extension was finished and it was time to knock through to our existing house. I found this very upsetting the place that I had shared time with my son was changing too quickly I wasn't ready for the change, my memories were being trashed, and some how I sat through endless banging, drilling, and workmen all over my home. I'd make tea by automation, being polite to their questions, but really wanting to scream at them to sod off and leave me alone.

Dust became my enemy it settled every where, and I had to spend endless hours cleaning, not only the dust, but the trash they left all over the front garden. One electrician even had the nerve to stand on a cushion on one of my dinning chairs in his dirty boots. It seemed they had no respect for me or my home. Under different circumstances I would had told them what I thought, but just weeks after my sons death I did not have the strength. Because both Nick and I were traumatized by the events over Easter neither were really aware of how the building was going, nor noticed very much, and in consequence we received and accepted very shoddy work in the finishing of our extension. The brick work was fine as were the foundations, but the rest is full of faults, there are some things I could have done better myself even though I'm not a builder. My brand new kitchen is already falling to bits. What saddens me is the fact that the main builder had known me for some years, knew what we had just been through and seemed to take advantage of our vulnerability. Now I have two spare bedrooms and no son to fill one of them with his things.

A policeman came to interview me a week or so after Edwards death, he needed a statement of events, and I had to go through the whole thing again in great detail, reliving each episode, including his life history and what sort of child he had been, that disturbed me for days, but I wasn't sleeping, when ever I did drop off I'd suffer night mares and Nick had to wake me when I started to cry out. I asked the policeman if they had found Edward's over night bag, as it was missing. He said he'd make inquiries, he contacted the Fair Mile and the Royal Berks Hospital both said no they had not seen his bag. The transport police were contacted they had not seen it, and we assumed Edward had either given it to someone, or had thrown it away.

August that year Nicks daughter in law gave birth to a beautiful little boy, their third child, he was born in the same hospital as Edward, and when I held him I could not stop the tears running from my eyes. The last baby I had held in that place had been Edward, and I could not control my sudden memory of that moment. I felt sorry it happened as it was the young couple's moment, and I did not want to mar their happiness.

Also in August 2002 I suddenly had a letter from a staff nurse of Ibsden ward at the Fair Mile to say they had Edward's bag would I like to collect it. The police collected it for me, it came in a transparent plastic bag from the Fair Mile, it had no name on it, and there was nothing inside to say whose bag it was. In it were changes of underwear, socks, a clean sweatshirt, tooth brush, wash things, an electric razor, a selection of Edward's CDs and a book. I wonder to this day how the Fair Mile after so many months and Edwards very brief stay on their ward knew that this was Edward's bag, especially when asked just after his death by the police for his bag, and they said they did not have it. How did they suddenly know this was Edward's bag after all that time and where had it been?

At the inquest in the October of 2002 the guy in the safari suit who turned out to be a nurse, gave evidence that Edward had asked to leave the hospital to collect some clothes from home, and when this nurse looked in Ed's bag he claimed all that was in the bag were a pair of under pants,

Edward may have been mentally ill but he would not have carried a large sports bag with just a pair of under pants in it, he was not suffering from dementure. This nurse said he asked Edward to wait until a nurse could go back to the house with him so he could collect some clothes? I have the bag up in the attic with the same things the nurse said were not there, still in it.

The policeman also took Edward's suicide note when I asked if it would be returned to me, he said he didn't know as it would be given to the coroner as evidence. I found this very upsetting, it was the last thing Edward ever gave me, and he handed it to me, because he wanted me to have it. At that time I had not found the courage to read it, at first I had an awful copy to read, that I was sent from the police each page along the bottom were black and unreadable. It took me four years to trace the original and have it returned.

That first year I had so much adrenalin in my body I needed to do things, after I decorated the completed extension, and did as much as I was able on renovating our home, I went out into the garden it had a patio, a walled herb garden Nick had built the first year we moved in, the rest was a square of what looked like field grass. I started to dig deep flower beds all along the back fence and around to one side, I dug and dug each day until I was exhausted, once dug I ferried endless wheel barrows full of gravel from the drive to make a path at the back of the flower beds by the fence, it took me months. Grief kept me going even when my body screamed out to stop. I didn't stop until Nick arrived home, on wet days I stayed in doors and cried myself stupid, as I wrote endless demented letters to everyone and anyone who had any connection to mental health. A kind of madness took over my head, I didn't want to see people or go any where. I went from being a person who loved to entertain and have friends and family round, or going visiting, to a recluse. Even after four years I still feel the same, when I do attend gatherings I never feel part of anything now, I sit on the edge of things, and keep my distance. Now it is only very few that get invited round. I've tried giving parties twice, once a couple of months after Nick and I married, and another for Nicks sixtieth Birthday, at both I worked myself silly doing endless things with food rather than finding time to talk to people.

The interviews and statements for the inquest seemed to go on forever, we were given three different dates each drifting into months ahead the first two were cancelled. My solicitor asked questions about what time did this happen? Or at what time was that? Wanting exact words people spoke, an in depth description of how Edwards injuries looked. I began to think that I should have had a tape recorder, camera, and stop watch, plus a note pad and pen, all over Easter, or that maybe I should always carry such things in case of an emergency. It was difficult to explain that when something really dreadful and unimaginable suddenly happens to your child, rational thinking does not exist the only thing that matters in that time is your child. What did it matter what time we left the Fair Mile, or what time Edward was allowed to walk out of the hospital to his death. The fact is he did walk out unnoticed whatever time we left or he left, when he should have been on suicide watch. But those sorts of questions were what he wanted answered, due to the other side's solicitors making a big thing out of the time things happened. The real fact is it happened due to their negligence no other facts are relevant.

I had a very strange relationship with my solicitor, part of me was very aware he was trying to help me, and doing his utmost for me, but another part found his detached mater of fact questions and comments very painful. My emotions had been ripped apart by what had happened to my son and the terrible sight I witnessed after his fall. I felt very raw and in so much pain, his cool approach was hard to deal with. Every phone call, letter brought the whole thing to the front of my mind and I was upset all over again. Those feelings would stay with me for days, and I found it hard to move away from that weekend, it stayed to the forefront of my mind for four years, I could not let my child rest.

My solicitor also felt I should look for compensation for psychological damage to me. I don't know what psychological damage is or if I am or was afflicted with it, I do know that I'm not the person I once was, and that I suffer all sort of things I never suffered before. I knew I wanted the Fair Mile to be aware of what they had done to Edward myself and my family. Because the solicitor was a no win no fee guy I had to have insurance in case we lost the case. He said my household insurance should cover solicitor's fees for damages to a person. When I contacted them we did have cover, but because at the time Edward was not living at home they would not help. I had to pay £200.00 and take out private insurance to cover me if I lost the case of physiological damages against me. I also had to sign a contract and if I broke this contract I would have been liable for any fees. I never realized until I found myself in this situation how evil the solicitors for the Berkshire Mental Health Trust would become, or how little the real truth had to do with law, I think that was the biggest shock, as I always felt the truth was what justice was about, but not when lawyers start playing with words.

I had to return to work in June as I was receiving no money and things were becoming financially very difficult. Nick around this time decided to stop smoking again, so it was better for me to be away for most of the day, as his temper was short and I was not fit enough emotionally to deal with it. At the time of returning to work I was a supervisor to five people in my department.

On my return, I found this very difficult, there was a harassment case going on with one member of staff against another, and because of my supervisory position I became embroiled with this. I found this really draining and difficult to deal with, though somehow I managed on the surface to carry on as normal, and no one realized just how stressed out I was. I also found it difficult to deal with trivial complaints and worries and small-mindedness of some my staff, I wanted to shout and scream at them, tell them what a real problem was really like. But I didn't I tried my best to calm things and sort things out. I found my concentration was not so good and simple tasks had become difficult. I dealt at the time with classified material and strict guidelines had to be carried out when booking such things in and out of the office. It took me twice as long to do things now and I found myself going over things several times, to make sure I was doing it correctly.

Due to the harassment case and I backing the victim, rather than moving the person accused, they moved the person that complained. I was also offered a different position in another department, at the same grad, but without staff. I accepted this and moved to a quieter area, and less stressful office. Though I had a steep learning curve in the new job, my fellow work colleges were far easier people to work with, and I managed to stay in the job for nearly three years before I put in for retirement. In the end it all became too much for me I feel far happier in my own home, and cope better with life on my own for most of the day.

Also in June 2002 I received a letter from a debt collector saying I owed them over £8,000. I was shocked and phoned them, it turned out to be a loan I had taken out on behalf of my younger sister by ten years, in May 1997 for half of that amount, and as far as I knew she was paying, but according to them no payment had been made since 1999, it had taken that long to trace me. I phoned my sister at work she said to send the letter onto her she would deal with it.

This I did and thought no more of it until September 2002 when I was sent a Court Order Notice if I didn't pay back all the money by a certain date, I would be taken to court. I went to pieces and Nick rang my sister's husband hoping to be able to talk to him man to man. Things went badly wrong, the call became abusive, and when my sister's partner said something about the way I was behaving over the inquest? Nick really lost his temper "Told him to fuck off." and put the phone down on him. I'm still not sure how one is meant to behave over an inquest. I in fact did very little apart from following the Coroner Officer's advice and my solicitors, so I'm not sure what it is I am suppose to have done, as I had never spoken to him about it. The only time I conversed with him was when he rang to say he wasn't coming to the funeral, and if had come it would only have been to support my sister.

The fall out between Nick and my sisters husband resulted with my sister putting a horrible message on the answer phone, and sending two terrible E-Mails, First one claimed I had never taken out a loan for her and that I had only attended my other sisters funeral in 1996 and gone back to the house after to see what insurance money she had left. She also claimed she had no sisters as we were both dead. The second E-Mail claimed that my sisters and my mother were always helping me out with bags of food and money when my children were small, this was not true, whatever the faults between Adrian and myself he had always been a good provider for his family, he had also lent them money some years before that was only partly paid back. She also claimed she had paid all the loan money back, a contradiction of her first E-Mail and that I had also made terrible accusation against a member of her family to one of her friends? What happened to me as a child I have never ever discussed with any member of my family, those I have spoken to about it besides medical persons, have been both my husbands, but never in detail to anyone. She must have heard about my past from someone else, but I have no idea who. This caused a great rift between my sister and I, sadly it turned my mother against me too.

My sister has recently received treatment for cancer and I have been in touch, though I still care what happens to her and worry about her health, I also miss her not being in my life, I can not remove her words from my head. It was only six month after my son's death and the words seemed to have cut very deeply into my mind, they seem to be tied up with my grief for Edward. Needless to say I am also still paying off this debt, something we can ill afford, when a Direct Debit is missed I am harassed by the credit company on the phone and by mail. I will probably be paying them until I die, as even though I did not have the money I signed the contract, so in law it's my debt. I find it really hard to think that someone I grew up with and love could have done this too me, when all I ever did was to try and help.

Also in September 2002 Jane and I were given the address of an organization called S.O.B.S. "Survivors of Bereavement by Suicide," we arranged to go along to one of the meetings. I'm not sure if it was too soon for us to attend after Edwards's death, or if it was the group, but it did not help us at all in fact we both felt worse. The group had been meeting for several years the same people with very few new people if any joining, and it was more like a group of jolly friends meeting up, than a self help group, all had lost someone but not that recently. They were very kind and listened to both Jane and I, one of the ladies as they were all women seemed quite aggressive in her response to us. She had lost her son a couple of years before. She could not understand why we stayed at the hospital and said she never went to the hospital to see her son. Neither did she go to his inquest and she told us we shouldn't go to Edward's, that we had no need to. She could not understand that we wanted to be there, even though we knew it was going to be stressful. I in fact was going to be called as a witness. I think she was still very troubled by her son's death and two years is not very long, her grief was still raw, but she did not seem to understand we all deal with death and grief in our own way, that there is no right or wrong way.

When we left we were so troubled by the meeting and so busy talking about how we felt, that we found our selves going down the M40 to London, and had to turn round at Stokenchurch. At that meeting one thing of interest came to light, both Jane and I admitted how we had both thought of taking our own lives just after Edward had died. We said we would not do it because of the rest of the family we couldn't put them through anymore. At that moment in time I really meant that and never dreamed that the following year I would forget those words.

NO TITLE

There must be a feeling that I can feel
There must be a place where I can deal with the hurt.
Many bruises have cut into me
Scaring the way on the road ahead that I must face.
So many times I have asked why
Why do I hurt by holding inside
I slowly watch, ripping pieces out of my mind.
Is there any truth?
Is there any way?
Could it be as simple as night and day?
Or am I running but making no headway.
Is there a need for haste?
Or am I running in the last race?
I'm reaching for a long lost case.
Or could writing this be a waste,
Because I feel the end is not far out of sight.
And I'm just reading more into black and white,
As for me I have a colouring book
Of feeling for all that's bright
And I know it would be dumb to lie
That when I see that spark in her eye
My mum and family, my love I can not deny.

INQUEST AND AFTER

After many meetings, endless letters, and phone calls the inquest date was set for the 22nd of October 2002 at 14-00hrs. This time it was not changed, neither my mother or sister came, my brother lived in Cromer and it was not possible for him to be there, but he had kept in constant touch by phone, since Edward first became ill. I did feel hurt by my mother not being there, or even contacting me after to find out how things went. But on reflection I don't ever remember my mother ever being there for me when I needed her, to me it always seemed to be the other way round, I being there for her, even when quite young. A dear friend whom I'd known since the sixties travelled from Cricklewood to be with me, I thought she was going to spend the night in Oxfordshire, but she returned home after the inquest and I was really touched by her being there for me and making such a long journey by train.

I had to meet up with my solicitor and barrister first at an address in Reading, Jack came with me. Nick stayed with Jane and met my friend from Cricklewood from the station and they made their way to the Coroners Court and met up with Adrian. After the brief meeting with my solicitor we made our way across Reading to the Coroners Court. The staffs from Ibsden Ward were there with Edward's last CPN and Dr. Mason none of them acknowledged me or any of the family, it was as if we were the enemy, not a family who had lost a loved one. Edwards's first consultant was there and offered his condolences, Edward's second consultant sat with him and away from the Ibsden staff.

The coroner explained the coroner's court was to find out what happened not to attach blame on anyone. The first witness was a young solider who had been sitting in his car when Edward fell and went to his aid and called an ambulance. I found this very distressing as it was the first time I had heard this statement. As I listened to the statements given by some of the Fair Mile staff, I wanted to correct their inaccuracies, but I was not allowed to comment, and had to sit and listen. They said he had had a meal with them, this I did not believe, and in my calculations he was with them for less than an hour, there was certainly no sign of food when we left, not even a smell of any. Why had Edward felt the need to travel to Reading to buy a sandwich if he had just eaten, he had brought a return ticket back to Cholsey, and must have intended to go back, but I believe the voices started up again, and that's what made him jump. The return ticket was in his wallet when the police returned it to me, I still have it. Why was the meal not recorded on his Observation Sheet, or mentioned in the autopsy report, he had not had enough time to digest what he may have eaten. In fact there was no sign of food having been eaten in the report.

They said he had asked to go home to collect some over night clothes, and when the nurse checked his bag, he claimed he did not have any wash things or a change of clothes, only a pair of under pants. I knew this to be a lie. The coroner also asked why he had not been sectioned as soon as he asked to go home, no one could give an answer.

When Dr. Mason was called I found out he had only

been working in with seriously mentally ill people for seven months, and had been left in charge of 164 patients over Easter weekend. He squirmed in his seat as he spoke, was still very arrogant and used long medical words to all his answers. He had miss diagnosed Edward, claiming he was suffering from drug induced psychosis, even though he had his medical records and his medical history. The post mortem had shown there were no drugs in Edwards's body or any alcohol. Dr. Mason claimed he had a superficial laceration to his neck and steri-strips applied, even though he had the doctor's report about internal and external sutures from the other hospital. He thought him to be a low risk for suicide and put him on a fifteen minute watch. They had his age down as 22 years when he was 20 years. It came out also that Edward's risk assessment was written up after his death and dated 01-04-02. They had him ticked for high risk age group (Elderly or young males) for suicide risk, but still thought him low risk, even though he had already made an attempt earlier that day. The risk management plan written up by the Fair Mile, states

"*To monitor mental state and observe and note any changes in mood, behaviour and interactions. To maintain Edward's safety to be nursed at level 3 of observations if need/or behaviour indicates increased risk - agitation, restlessness, increased withdrawal and preoccupation. To administer prescribed medication and monitor effects and any side effects. To offer individual time to establish a rapport and trust to allow Edward to discuss any concerns he may have regarding his treatment plan. To liaise closely all findings and any concerns to the medical team."*

All well and good apart from the fact it was dated after Edward's death, this was brought up in the inquest by the Coroner as was the question of medication, Dr. Mason was asked why Edward was not given any medication on his arrival, and why it was not going to be given until 22-00hrs on the evening of his admittance. Dr. Mason gave a long medical detailed comment about why, that few understood, but could not give any real reason as to why Edward was to wait that long for medical treatment.

When Edward's new consultant from the Fair Mile was called he said it was a preventable death that Edward's life could have been saved if he had been put on a higher watch. He also said that even though he was on leave he had asked to be notified if any of his patients were admitted over Easter weekend. Staff of Ibsden Ward claimed they had phoned him, but it appears they only phoned once, when they say he was not available. It also came out that at the beginning of March the Berkshire Mental Health Trust had brought in a new operation for keeping watch on patients and if Ibsden Ward had been using this Edward would not have been able to walk out. It also came to light that two other patients had already walked out unnoticed that day, yet they did not lock the ward or keep a good watch on the rest of the patients until after Edward walked out. The other two people were brought back safely that evening. It also came to light that the ward had the correct amount of staff on duty, so their shoddiness can not be put down to staff shortages.

The CPN when she gave her evidence was very defensive and gave as many digs as she could against me. What her problem was with me I will never know, to me my son's mental health was what mattered and if my need to talk to her about him interfered with her tiny little world then tough. When I gave my evidence the solicitors for the Berkshire Mental Health Trust made a big thing about the time we left Edward at the Fair Mile. "I put it to you that you left the ward at 16-30" their barrister demanded from me, I said it was possible, though I know for sure I didn't, but saw no point in arguing over time. At that time it had not registered the staff had written up times that did not correspond with my times or the families, and that's why it became such an issue with the solicitors.

I feel the staff doctored everything to cover up the failings that led to my son's death, and no one will convince me otherwise. I'm no detective but just reading through their paper work explains it all. I don't believe he was given a bed, food, or was on any particular watch, I suspect he walked out not long after we left, and no one noticed until his father rang to see if he had settled in. His notes being missing for two weeks, gave them time to have a plausible story and written notes to confirm their story. They claimed they found his notes in the nurse's desk drawer on Ibsden ward? Why on the day they were looking for his notes did they not check that drawer. They may have got away with some of it if they had not dated the notes incorrectly.

Five hours after the start of this inquest the Coroner declared Edward died "While unbalanced of the mind aggravated by lack of care." My solicitor said lack of care was not recognisable in law, what it really meant was " Death while unbalance of the mind aggravated by negligence" For some strange reason some of the Fair Mile staff cheered, and Dr. Mason happily went out of the court and started talking and laughing on his mobile phone. I think they thought some sort of blame was going to be put on to one of them. But their lack of respect at that moment for my son, myself and my family will always stay with me.

After the inquest my solicitor started to put a case together for physiological damage, Jack declined to be involved right from the beginning. He was in a terrible state at that time, the death of his brother hit him really badly, and he was very unwell. Jack and Edward had been good mates, they watched rugby and football together, and they played and discussed computer games. They argued good naturedly about their different life styles, and out look on life. After Edwards death Jack had trouble trying to keep his shop going due to almost having a break down after what he had witnessed that

Easter, he continued to try and work, but he was not well enough and his heart was not in it. The shop went into liquidation in December that year, the receivers going in on Christmas Eve, and Jack went missing. He was found in the dark up at Edward's grave in tears, telling Edward what had happened. The financial impact on him and Louise due to his brothers death was tremendous, they almost lost their home, and they struggled for a long time, Jack was out of work for some months, but was not eligible for any help or benefits, due to being self employed for a few months. Yet he's worked none stop since the age of sixteen and paid tax and insurance all the time. Both sides of the family were helping out as much as we were able. Now they both work as many hours as they can, both still afraid of being in that situation again. The thought of going to court was too much for Jack, his mental state at that time was very fragile.

Jane at first said she would become involved, but after her first interview with the solicitor, she with drew. We were all very vulnerable at that time and the questions asked by the solicitor were very painful. She has always been a very sensitive person and like Jack she was very fragile at that time, she came to me in tears and said she could not cope with the solicitor, she found him too hard and cold. He was quite young and I felt he had spent most of his time dealing with physical claims, and had no idea how to approach those with emotional damage. Jane hid her grief from me most of the time, doing her best to stay strong for me.

She found it difficult to cry and felt bad because the tears would not come, and she thought something was wrong with her. The fact was she was so traumatized by the whole weekend, she was in shock, which lasted for two years or more. There were twelve years between Jane and Edward and she was like a second mother to him. He used to talk to her about most things, and discuss films and books they had seen or read.

The first Christmas after Edwards's death, in a daze she walked out of a surfing, and skaters, shop in Reading that Edward liked with a sweat-shirt for Edwards Christmas present. She was arrested and given a five-year caution, she was so numb and shocked by what she had done, that she did not say anything about what she had been through. She never told me until several months after, when I heard I felt so upset for her, and wished she had rung me at the time. I tried writing to the chief constable of the Thames Valley police explaining the circumstances, but he said there was nothing he could do, once the custody officer gave a caution it could not be changed. I did try the custody officer but he didn't even bother to reply. It saddens me that she has this hanging over her, she certainly did not deserve it, there is no one more honest and straight than Jane. My daughter has suffered many problems since the death of her brother and I worry about both my remaining children far more than I ever did. I panic now if I can't reach them on the phone, or I don't hear from them regularly.

After Edward died Jane had a very strong need to visit a Medium, she wanted to see if it was possible to contact Edward, and make sure he was alright. She asked me to accompany her when she found one. I wish I could have felt the same as her, but I'm very sceptical. The Medium I believe was genuine, and not out to make money, though she was only expecting Jane, she never charged any more for me. We sat in a semi darkened room in her home, in Reading, it was very quite. Jane and I sitting close together she was facing us, quite close but not in touching distance. Her voice was soft and there was an air of peace around us. A couple of people came to her first an elderly dapper man and an elderly woman holding a small white dog. I could put both to a member of my family, but did not say very much. Both Jane and I had agreed we would not give any information freely before we went in.

Then she said "I have a young man here beside me, he has a message for you." and she looks towards me " he say's he's very sorry to have put you through so much, he did not mean to hurt you."

She asked if that meant anything and I confirmed it did. She continued with," This person has not passed over that long ago, he's having a few problems staying with me. Just a minute he's trying to show me something, it's a sandwich, not cheese more like the pressed type of cheese, the sort that's individually wrapped. I've never had this before, does it mean anything to you?" I confirmed it did, as Edward only liked cheese slices in a sandwich. She said he wanted us to know he was alright, that he had been trying to let us know, but we never understood his signs.

She then said again looking at me, " He say's you did the right thing, not going into the room, but staying at the door, that he didn't want you to go in. Do you understand that." Again I confirmed that I did by now tears were running down my face, and Jane and I were holding hands.

She continued with " He say's he likes the yellow flowers. Does that mean anything." I shook my head so did Jane we both pondered over the flowers we had at his funeral, but there was no predominant yellow. The medium explained that it may mean something when we think of it later. It did, the evening before a friend had brought round a flower display, and her daughter was doing a flower-arranging course. It was just before Christmas and the table arrangement she gave me, was tones of gold that included yellow roses.

She said he liked a drink, that he was helping others that passed over, and had befriended the boy that drowned. Again this meant nothing, until about a month later, there was a report in the local paper about an inquest of a fourteen year old that had drowned in the Thames not far from Selsea Place, I had forgotten about that, until I read the report.

I still don't know what to believe it certainly surprised me, I can't say if it was just a lucky guess on the Mediums part, but then how did she make so many correct assumptions, even if she was able to read our body language and notice other things about us. She ended with "I think you need to give him a rest for a while before you try and contact him again, he's very new at this." We've not been again, we have spoken of it but I'm afraid if it didn't pick up on so many things a second time, it would destroy the comfort I found in the first meeting, even if I'm still not really sure if I believe it was him.

But I have digressed, Adrian at first was going to go through with the court case with me but in the end could not, like me he was badly damaged by what we had been through that Easter weekend, he required counselling and constant visits to his GP over the next few years as I did. I had signed the contract and had only one way to go, the next few years turned into a night mare, I was constantly reminded what had happened and was unable to see if I could move on, I kept reliving the whole thing over and over, even when I did not want to. I was going through it not for money, but for my son and my family all who had been damaged by the inefficiency and lack of interest of the Fair Mile Hospital. I wanted the Fair Mile to remember what they had done, and try and stop it happening to someone else's child, hitting them financially I felt was the one way they would possibly not forget.

In January 2003 I had a health check at work, this showed I had very high blood pressure, and I was advised to visit my GP. On my next visit as I was attending the surgery regularly since Edwards death. My doctor checked my blood pressure, I had several other tests. An ECG showed my heart had a problem, and I ended up going to hospital to see a heart specialist after several more tests I was told I had Cardiomyopathy (heart failure). I was told the left side of my heart was enlarged and that the left ventricle was very floppy and not closing fully. They had no idea what had caused it, and that there was no cure all they could do was give me medication to slow the deterioration down. I was sure it was caused by stress but no one would confirm this. I read prolonged stress could cause high blood pressure, and that in turn could damage the heart or kidneys, or lead to diabetes. I've never smoked, never been a heavy drinker, eat sensibly, and do a lot of walking. There's only one thing that had happened to me recently to raise my blood pressure so badly that was my son's death. Since my divorce and before Edward became ill I had been happy and stress free. Though the hospital told me things would not change and my heart would deteriorate over time, my last check at the hospital, showed there had been improvement in the ventricle, the consultant was surprised and happy for me but could not explain why it had improved, so though the left side of my heart is still enlarged, the left ventricle is functioning better than it was. I'm pretty sure I know why, my stress levels have become less as time goes on.

In 2003 Nick and I also went to see a solicitor about making wills, it became so complicated due to us only living together and both having children, that we gave up the idea. It seems it was far easier if we were married, so Nick asked me to marry him. He had asked me several times before, but we never really bothered we were happy as we were. But since Edwards's death we had become aware how fragile life is, and we wanted things safe for the other if either of us should die. Out of respect for Nick's children we decided only to have both our children their partners, and grandchildren at the registry office. But that proved too difficult for Nick's children and neither of them attended. I know it was a very painful time for Nick and I felt his hurt, we married in Wantage Town Hall on the 19th June 2003 with just Jane, Jack, Louise and a couple from the village. We looked a sad little affair in such a vast hall, but Nick and I went to Paris for a week after and recuperated.

A week or so before the marriage I sent a letter to a member of Nicks family who had been upset the last time we had seen them. I tried to explain that we had not been in touch very much due to myself being with drawn since Edward's death, that none of it was Nicks fault. Whatever I said though not meant, it caused offence, and a phone message said I was never to enter their home again or see any of their children.

If this happened now I would go round and speak to

them, to try and find out what I had written that offended them, and talk it through. But at the time I was very irrational still trying to accept Edward was dead, and that he was not going to walk through the door one day, or suddenly be on the phone. I had a copy of the letter sent and I reread it but could not see what I had done wrong. It was meant to be a caring letter, one of reassurance, but some how it went terribly wrong. I tried to phone, but only spoke on the answer phone, that resulted in an angry phone call to Nick, who by now was very angry with me, and life in general.

I stood in the kitchen for sometime crying, when a strange calmness came over me, I had no thought in my head, but the real need for escaping the shit life I seemed to be in. My youngest son was somewhere and I needed so much at that moment to take him in my arms I wanted to be out of the pain that sat inside me every day. I took the anti-depressants I'd been taking since Edward's death, and put one in my mouth, swallowed a mouthful of water, and took another one, I continued in that fashion. It was like I was standing outside my body just watching myself swallow those pills, I had had most of the packet by the time Nick came into the room. He ranted at me more in fear than anything, and yelled "What are you doing."

"I want out, I want oblivion" I yelled back "I don't want this shit and pain any more."

Nick phoned our GP after grabbing the pills off me

and then bundled me into the car and took me to A&E in Oxford. There I was hitched up to a heart monitor, they asked me how many tablets I had taken I said the first number that came into my head, as I had no idea how many I'd taken. My heart was racing I could feel it pumping in my chest, I was wheeled into the resuscitation room, they were convinced my heart was going to stop, and they kept asking me if I had any chest pains. Nick left me there too stressed and upset to stay. I remained hitched up to the monitor all night fortunately my heart rate began to slow over the night. Sometime in the early hours I was wheeled into the same over night ward Edward had been in. In the morning Jane came to see me she was in tears and I felt so mean to do that to her. I hated myself for giving Nick and Jane so much stress and pain, but at the same time I felt so over whelmed by my own pain I was unable to think of others and found I could not cope, though I felt very selfish for putting them both through so much worry.

I was finding it difficult to be there for others, yet I felt that was my roll in life and what everyone expected of me, to be the strong one, the one that solved and helped everyone, that I never needed anyone to ever be strong for me, that I was always there. It's a roll impressed on me from such an early age I can't shake it off. Yet at that time I felt the need for someone to be strong for me, to take all the responsibility away from me for awhile, for someone else to take on that roll.

Sadly Nick started to smoke again that evening and I blamed myself for this for a long time. I had to talk to a psychiatric nurse when I explained things to her, what had happened to my son, how I felt and how I never meant any harm writing the letter, she said I was suffering from Post Traumatic Stress Disorder. This resulted in my seeing a psychiatrist once a month and a medical psychologist every week for almost a year. They helped me see things from another point of view, and I was shown how to deal with the flash backs I was getting. Though it did not take away the pain, or many of my fears it has helped me to deal with them, and made me realize it is all right to do things for just me, that I don't have to put everyone else first. Though I do have to remind myself of that one every so often.

In September 2003 my mother had a massive stroke, my brother phoned me after seeing mum and advised me not to visit her as she would not know me, and he felt it would be too upsetting for me, and that I had been through enough. I had hopped she would recover and be able to attend Jack and Louise's wedding that was arranged for early October. I felt it would be a good time for mum, my sister and I to put things on a happier setting.

But sadly mum died before the wedding, so my sister and her husband never bothered to attend the wedding. Though they had accepted the invitation this did cause the young couple a problem, as everything had been catered and paid for by the time they let them know they were not coming. I travelled to Essex with Nick and Jane for mum's funeral, I was still very numb and found it difficult to relate the funeral to my mother. In fact I still don't really feel I have grieved for her, I seemed to have blocked it out. I did not go back to the reception after the funeral service in the chapel. My sister's words were going round in my head, about me only going back after the funeral of my sister to see if she had left any money. Since that comment I have never gone back to any receptions after attending some ones funeral, I don't think I ever will, unless it is one that I have to arrange.

In January 2004, I found myself in hospital again, this time because I had damaged the cartilage on my left knee in November 2003. I was in a great deal of physical pain, it was so sharp with certain movements that it took my breath away, and at times made me involuntary cry out, this I found very embarrassing especially when out shopping etc. Then just before Christmas as I crossed the road my knee gave way completely. It felt like an elastic band in the back of my leg had snapped, I fell to the ground in great pain and discovered I could not walk. I was on crutches for months, before and after the operation. It wasn't until June that year that I began to feel pain free. That year I also had day admittance for an angiogram of my main arteries and heart, this showed my arteries were healthy, so that had not caused my heart problem. I'd always been very fit physically so I found all of this very taxing. I had ignored my body for so many years now suddenly it was letting me know I needed to care for it.

The court case drifted on eating up my years, stopping me even trying to lay Easter 2002 to rest. The solicitors from the Berkshire Mental Health Trust, said I could not be traumatized because I did not see Edward fall. This really upset me, as I knew he had been conscious after his fall and trying to talk to the paramedics and at the hospital before he was heavily sedated, even now it hurts because I was not by his side to comfort him. I see him fall as I drift off to sleep most nights and wake with a start. I can't watch any one on T'V' or a film jump or fall from a great height any more. I also have a fear of heights now, something that never effected me before, I've travelled over the Alps and the Pyrenees in a car without any fear, now suddenly I really start to panic, I sweat, my heart races and I'm near to tears when ever I am near to the edge of something now. When in the Lake District and once last year in the car close to the edge of the road with a drop to the sea, I had these feelings and found myself crying out.

Next they claimed that I had been given counselling before I went into to see Edward when we arrived at the Royal Berks Hospital after his fall? By whom or when they never said, I certainly can not remember any counselling, all the medical personnel's I saw had only concern for my son, as I would have expected it to be. Any way this counselling I am suppose to have had made them claim I was not shocked by the sight of him? They also claimed I was not with him for long at the hospital after his fall, and that I did not go into ICU when he was there, but only stayed at the door? So I had to try and remember how many times I went into see him in the Intensive Care Unit, and how long I stayed with him each time? There was also some big thing about the time laps between Edward falling and I getting to the Royal Berks Hospital, I kept saying we left for the hospital as soon as we heard, and we did not even know if it was Edward at that time. What should have been straight forward, became more and more complicated as the Royal Berks Mental Health Trust tried to wriggle out of taking any responsibility.

I had to see an expert witness for both sides, for my solicitor in 2004 I had to see a psychiatrist who practiced in a hospital in Manchester. She had read all my notes and knew what had taken place, she said she did not want me to go through all that, but to explain how I felt about it all. She talked about the depression I had suffered over the years, about my childhood. I was with her for about forty-five minutes, her report said as I had suffered with depression she had expected Edward's death to have made me depressed. That I had been traumatized by the events of that day, and she fully expected some of the effects to stay with me for the rest of my life.

The expert witness for the other side I had to travel

to Harley Street in London in 2005, this psychiatrist was not practicing medicine any more, she only worked as an expert witness, and she was referred to as Royal Berks Mental Health Trusts big guns, by the doctor I saw in Manchester at a meeting sometime later. This person kept me in her office for two and a half hours without a break. She claimed she knew nothing about Edward, so she made me go through things in fine detail, starting with Edwards's childhood. She didn't take any notes as the other doctor had, she just wrote down odd words on a note pad now and again. Then she wanted to know my history, I went through everything, she had my medical notes in front of her, and for someone who had not read any information about me, she found all the bouts of depression I had very quickly in the notes and asked what caused my depression on such dates going back into the seventies.

Apart from post natal depression and a miserable marriage I could not help her, as I don't remember why I was depressed all those years ago or even if there was a reason. As I was about to leave, she had already terminated the interview and I was standing ready to go to the door, she mentioned that I must be nervous about the coming court case. I confirmed that I was, and she asked if I was worried about the cost. I explained that I had a no win no fee solicitor, so it should not be a problem. She said how much you think it is so far. I told her I had no idea, and she mentioned some large sum of money and laughed as she said that makes your sisters debt seem very little.

When her report arrived I was totally shocked by the mistakes, she claimed that Edward became ill due to Nick and I marrying? Ed died in 2002, we married in 2003. There were mistakes all the way through it, with many contradictions none of the history was correct, and she used the chat about the cost of my solicitor in the text of the report as if I had discussed it with her during our interview. She said I would have been depressed even if Edward had not died, she quoted from various medical books as proof. She also claimed that I had not been traumatized by the events of that day. For the first time in my life I was made to feel guilty for suffering with depression on and off in my life and seeking help from my GP I understood the stigma others are made to feel by the attitude of someone.

This report was damning and the barrister for our side who had thought we had a 60% chance of winning against the Berks Mental Health Trust 40% of winning, suddenly reversed the figures. Even though I went through the report paragraph by paragraph writing out all inaccuracies, this report was seen as some sort of bible that could only be true, and the barrister was sure we did not stand a chance. The fight was knocked out of me if I couldn't have faith and trust of those suppose to be on my side, and they believed this woman over me, to me I had already lost the case. I have since written to this Expert Witness when I discovered she was a supporter of Rethink, I asked her why she wrote what she did. I did receive a reply where she claims she agrees with the other expert witness, and her results were not adverse to my claim? Shame my learned barrister miss read it, as did many others including myself!

In September 2005 the Royal Berkshire Mental Health Trust offered £60,000 to end the case, and I accepted. Out of that £40,000 was paid to my solicitor and I received £20,000. £2,500.00 of that was for Edwards pain from the time he fell to the time he was sedated? I gave my children money and some to Nicks, we paid off some debts. We brought some new things for our selves and I brought many gifts and treats for others, and Nick and I had a weeks holiday. The money meant nothing to me it wasn't my son, I found it an insult to put a price of £20,000 on my messed up life and that of a loving young man, who did not deserve to die, certainly not the terrible way he did. But I hope hitting them in the pocket makes them remember Edward, and they think twice when some other person who has attempted to take their own life, enters their hospital as a place of safety.

Dr. Mason now works with elderly people? Adrian complained to the GMC about him, but they did nothing. I've found out since that he was a suspended surgeon before he started to work for the Fair Mile as a psychiatrist. A mother of five had died after he had used laser surgery on her, and that another patient had also died after surgery and that is why he was suspended and he had been disciplined for drinking while on duty, and also for watching Manchester United play football, when on call rather than answering his bleeper. That was the arrogant doctor who had allowed my son to walk out of a place of safety, because he did not bother to look at Edwards's notes or listen to his family, but made his own conclusions incorrectly.

I've been asked several times if I ever feel anger towards Edward. I never have to me it was the illness that led to Edwards death. He did not want to die. My anger is with the people I trusted to keep him safe from his illness. Big anger towards the independent doctor on his first Mental Health Review Tribunal that Christmas 2000, if he had done things correctly and spent time interviewing Edward and read his notes, his section would not have been discharged. He would have been moved to Section Three if he continued to not comply with his medication. He would have remained in hospital receiving treatment until he was well enough to come home, where I could have continued to care for him. Instead of him leaving hospital while still unwell and living in that awful bed and breakfast.

I have anger with "care in the community" because his care fell very short of what he should have received, because my son was an "Overlap". I feel terrible anger towards Dr. Mason and his arrogance and lack of interest, I have anger towards a CPN who fell very short of her care towards my son, and froze out those who really cared about him. Who also tried to lay blame on me at the inquest, this I find unforgivable.

There are dedicated people out there as well as types like his last CPN and Dr. Mason, I met them too, both his consultants at the Warnford and Fair Mile, Ginny the social worker who helped out when Edward was in limbo, Dan his warden in Selsea Place, and his first CPN also Rob his named nurse at the Warnford. Thank goodness there are such people.

I feel terrible anger at the Berkshire Mental Health Trust for putting me though four years of needless pain, because they were too mean to admit the damage caused, and for allowing the lies being made against me by their solicitors. It makes a mockery of the letter of apology they sent me.

I'm pleased the Fair Mile has at last closed, the old building is a listed one, there's talk of turning it into apartments. What a place to choose to live…its walls crying for all those poor souls that have lost their lives over many years. I hope the new hospital in Reading has wards that are for the age group of sixteen to twenty-five for seriously mentally sick, they should not be put in a ward full of older people, their needs are different and they should not be ignored. But sadly any hospital is only as good as the people working in it, if those from Ibsden Ward are still employed there then I pity those in their care.

Edward would have been twenty-five in November

2006. When the consultant first diagnosed paranoia schizophrenia, I had asked him what the out look was for my son. He explained there were degrees of the illness. That some only ever have one psychotic episode and never have any more. That others suffer several bouts up to around the age of twenty-five, and sadly others had it very severely and would have psychotic episodes through out their lives. He felt Edward was in the middle, and that by thirty he would be over the psychosis, and though he would be different to the person he once was with medication he would be able to live a normal life, and that he knew many that did, and went onto hold down jobs and have families of their own. Thanks to Ibsden Ward and Dr. Mason my son never had the chance to find out. The Human Rights Act, Article Two, states that a suicidal person in an institution IE hospital has the right to life, as did my son, they took away his right to life.

I still have bad moments, and times when I am still irrational. The bouts of depression now are much deeper. It's like I fall into a whirlpool and am being sucked down. Before Edward died being in that whirlpool I could just manage to keep my head above the water, and cling to the edge. Now I feel as if I'm in the very centre, the suction is much stronger, and water at times washes over my head. I feel it is a very thin thread that keeps me afloat, my senses seem far more acute when I feel like this, and I hurt all over.

When on a long journey I can't stop that Easter

creeping back into my mind. I go over events they play in my head like a DVD, moments are paused as I try to work out why, or what could have been done differently. I still find it unbearable to think of the pain and fear he must have felt after his fall, before he was sedated, and I wasn't with him. I worry that after he jumped, he may have changed his mind as he did earlier that day when he tried to end his life with a knife, but there was no going back the second time. These thoughts are often with me in the early hours of the morning, or as I said when travelling long distances. Some nights I still can not drop off to sleep my brain is full of Edward and I go over events in my head, at these times silent tears run down my face.

I have learnt from this awful tragic event too, my trust in doctors and the law is very poor now. I feel money is not the answer to happiness, neither are possessions, but peace of mind is. I feel the most important things in my life are the people around me, family, and good friends whom I love and care about. Without these people my life would be very poor, life is very fragile none of us know how long we have with each other, and I want to make the most of those I hold dear to me, and hopefully live a stress free life from now on.

I try very hard now to think of the positive things in my life, I live in a decent house with a garden made out of love in a pleasant down land village. My home has a great view of the rolling downs, where horses, sheep and cows graze. I have two loving children, Nick's two children and their families whom I care about, beautiful grand children on both sides – also a few good friends whom I feel close to.

A husband who accepts me for who I am and has no expectations of me, he's also my best friend. He has had a rough time of it, I'm not the same person he first met, and I've changed. He finds me sad at times because I don't laugh so much, and I take things far more seriously now.

There have been good times, lovely things have happened over the four years too. Jack and Louise married on the 11th of October 2003, and Nick's son married on the 19th of June 2004, both lovely weddings with beautiful brides, and a happy family occasion for everyone. Then on the 7th of July 2005 Louise gave birth to an adorable baby boy. He's a lovely and very special child to our family, he's given us a new beginning, his dear little face is always bright with smiles, with his whole life in front of him, full of innocence and trust, and he gives us something to marvel at as we watch him develop.

Edward will never be forgotten and will always be missed, there's a place in my heart that is there just for him. There's a pain there whenever I think of him, his memories I hold close to that spot, and often through the unshed tears now I can also think of him with a smile as I remember many treasured times we shared. On every family occasion he is still deeply missed, there is an empty place where he should be. But laughter has returned in our lives now, so I will end with one of Edwards lighter poems, and you can share his sense of fun with me.

BIKES

When you're out and about
You better watch out
For those fast bikes that zoom about.
Because I knew a man called Pete
Who had a bike run over his feet.
Outraged by this uncalled for attack
He bloody well hit back!
He gave it an almighty boot
And the bike went toot.
The cyclist was scared he had to have a pee
And Pete just went 'errr' and kicked him in the knee.
Pete's feet have finally got better.
But as for the bike it went to the wrecker.

Berkshire Healthcare NHS
NHS Trust

Church Hill House
51-52 Turing Drive
Bracknell
Berkshire
RG12 7FR

28th April 2002

Dear Miss Courtney,

On my own behalf and on the behalf of Berkshire Healthcare NHS Trust, I wish to offer my apologies to you and your family for the treatment received by your son, Edward Best, at the Fair Mile Hospital in March 2002.

The Trust accepts that the treatment provided to your son by the hospital fell below an acceptable standard. The Trust admits, with hindsight, that the appropriate observation level should have been level 2 rather than 3. In addition, the Trust admits that there was failure to keep Edward on the premises. As a result of those admitted failings, it is accepted that Edward's death on 1st April 2002 may possibly have been prevented.

I would like to express my deepest sympathies to you and your family. I can confirm that an internal inquiry into Edward's death was conducted by the Trust. I understand that the Director of Nursing and the Senior Nurse at Fair Mile, visited you with a copy of the draft report. You were able to comment on the report and it is being amended to reflect your views. Once the final report is published, a copy will be provided to you. It is my fervent wish and intention that lessons will be learned from your son's death to reduce the risk of such a tragedy occurring again in the future.

Yours sincerely

Chief Executive.

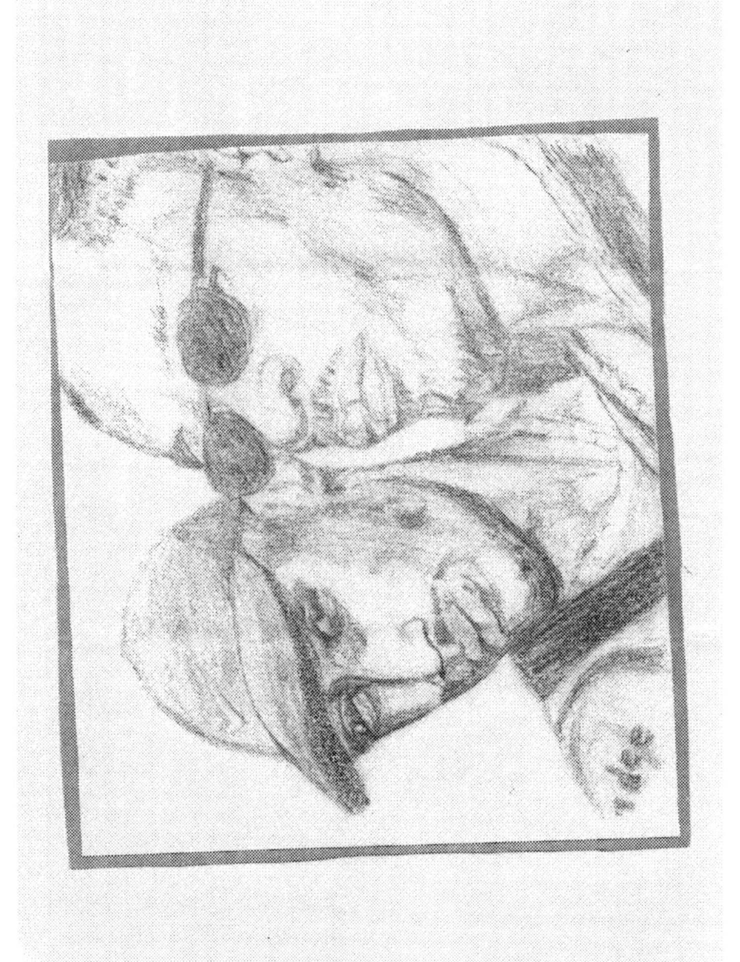

Edwards drawing
completed age 12

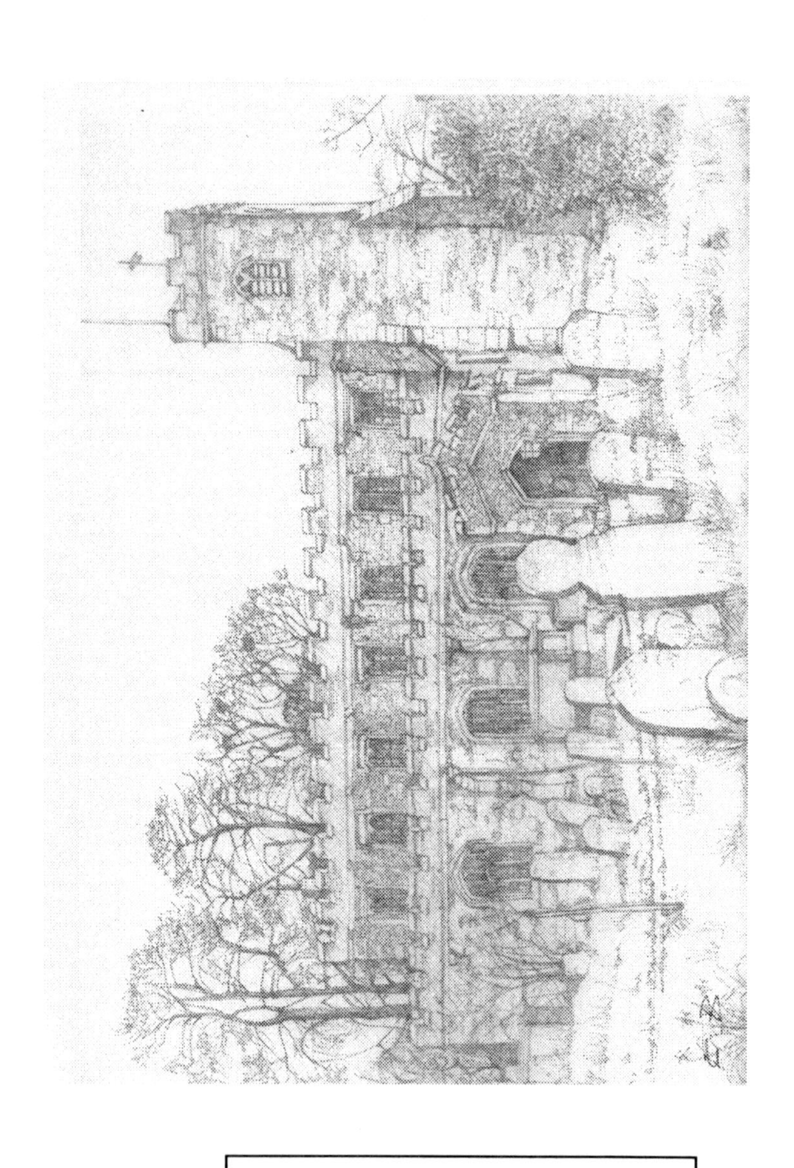

Edwards drawing for art A level 2001

Printed in the United Kingdom
by Lightning Source UK Ltd.
121037UK00001B/79